KETO DIET FOR BEGINNERS

THE ULTIMATE GUIDE FOR LOSING WEIGHT AND TRANSFORMING YOUR BODY WHILE EATING DELICIOUS MOUTHWATERING FOOD

JESSE RYAN FROM KETO LIFE MASTERY

❀ Created with Vellum

NOTE FROM THE AUTHOR

Hi there,

We all know the troubles that come along with starting a new diet. Hopefully, with the recipes found in the following pages, I can help you "ease" into the Keto diet. The Keto diet was the last "diet" I've had to follow. I hope that this, too, becomes the case for you.

- Jesse from Keto Life Mastery

JOIN OUR THRIVING KETO COMMUNITY!

Join our FREE Facebook Group and get The Keto Starter Kit: delicious swaps, shopping lists and keto cheat sheets!

Click here to join: https://www.facebook.com/groups/382874099248857/

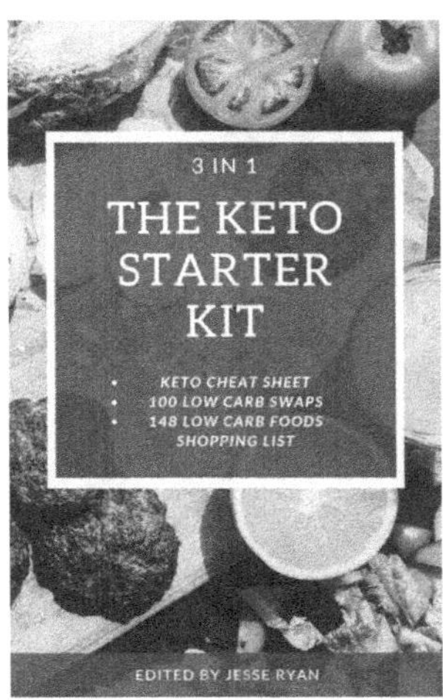

INTRODUCTION

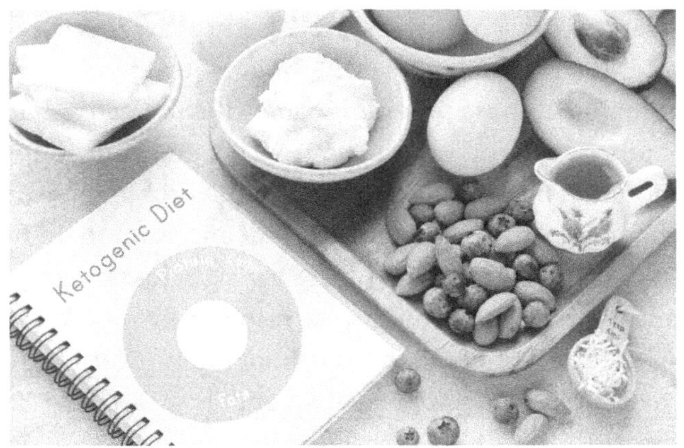

Do you ever feel like your body is working against you when you are trying to lose weight? You know the drill: find a diet, follow it and change your life accordingly. Faced with the dilemma of losing weight, you either choose a do-it-yourself, DIY plan; or, you decide to let someone else control your fate i.e. Jenny Craig or Weight Watchers. Once you've made that decision, you follow the plan exactly as directed; but in the end, you don't lose the same amount of weight as other people in your group. You are trying as hard as the next person, but still nothing.

Is It More Than Just Losing Weight?

Maybe it isn't just the issue of losing weight anymore. Perhaps there is something else that you want to change. For example, do you feel terrible after you eat? Do you feel like you are putting the wrong kind of fuel in your tank because you just don't have the get-up-and-go that other people have? Furthermore, do you spend more time feeling sick then your friends and family? The motivation to exercise or to participate inactivities is just not there, because you are always so tired. This is the way I began to feel, so I went looking for answers.

The Big Business of Losing Weight

In today's world, losing weight has become big business. There are organizations and companies like Weight Watchers, Noon, Nutri-System and Jenny Craig that will hold your hand through the process. Yet none of these programs come cheap. The primary goal of these programs is for you to open your wallet and contribute a never-ending amount of money in order to solve the problem for you.

But what if you're an independent soul and want to do-it-yourself (DIY)? Is it possible for a person to DIY a weight loss program?

The answer to that question is a resounding yes! You can help yourself with the right book and our book: <u>Keto Diet for Beginners: The Ultimate Guide for Losing Weight and Transforming Your Body While Eating Delicious, Mouth-Watering Food</u>, is the right book for you.

Looking for Answers

Can there possibly be another way to lose weight and transform your body that actually works? Wanting to answer this question, I turned to film for answers. While doing my research, I came upon a movie star-ringMeryl Streep titled: "Do No Harm".This movie is about a very young boy who is diagnosed with epilepsy. The doctors cannot find a medical cure to help the boy. All they can offer is an intensive brain surgery that may or may not work. Meryl Streep, who plays the mother of this boy, is desperate to find a cure. So, she concentrates on the research found in medical books and she comes across it: The Ketogenic diet

With some struggle, Meryl Streep finally gets her son to John Hopkins where he is put on the Ketogenic diet and after being on it for three years, he never has another seizure. In fact, in the US, many adults and children have been cured of their epileptic seizures just by going keto. I love that film!

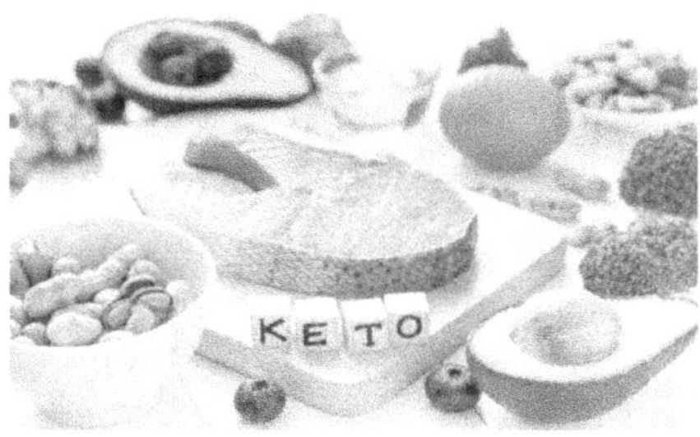

The Keto Diet is Born

Developed in the 1920s by Drs. Stanley Cobb and W.G. Lennox of Harvard Medical School and Dr. Russel M. Wilder of the Mayo Clinic, the Ketogenic diet has been found to help people who are diabetic or overweight. Many people have chosen the Keto diet just to IMPROVE their overall health, let alone lose weight.

The Life-changing Keto Diet

The Ketogenic diet is not a difficult diet to follow, yet it is life changing. Developed and sanctioned by many in the medical community, the Keto diet profoundly changes the way you feel physically, by metabolically changing your body's way of burning fat and producing energy.

In the age of the Mediterranean diet or the Zone diet, how can a protocol that was created in the 1920s be such a popular diet of the 21st century? Is it because you can eat hamburgers and steak? Is it because you don't have to count calories or points? Or is it because you just feel pretty darn good about what you're eating?

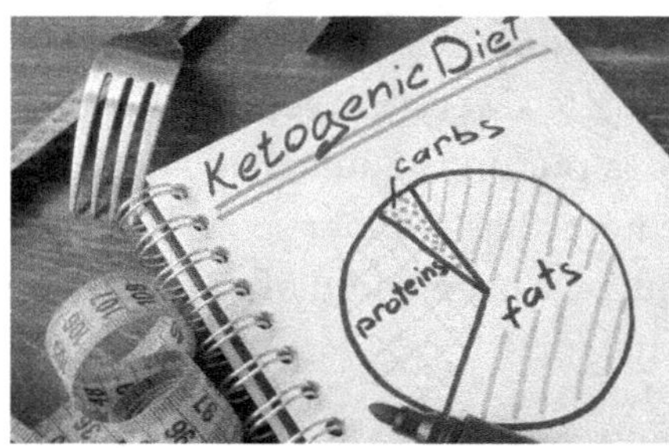

I've been successfully following the Ketogenic diet for a while now, and I am rarely ever hungry. In fact, with a little information about the Keto diet, I learned to conquer cravings and stick to the plan. Doing this has made me feel healthier than I ever have before. Feeling good and not having to be stressed with counting points or calories, was very effective in helping me to stay on track and follow this new healthy way of eating.

How Does It Work?

The Ketogenic way of eating is a diet where you get most of your calorie intake from protein and healthy fats. The basic formula for the Keto diet is: 70% fat, 20% protein and 5% carbohydrates. That might sound hardcore, but with a little bit of help from this book, you will learn how to plan meals and make choices that fit the Keto diet.

The reason for following this formula is that it sets in motion a new way for your body to get energy and burn fat. Primarily the body runs on glucose. When you eat carbs, the body takes the calories from carbs and turns them into energy – bypassing the fat that you have stored in your body. When you follow the food plan on the Keto diet, you recalibrate your body and the way it burns fat. When you put less carbohydrates in your body, your body will seek out your stored fat for energy. This produces acids that are called ketones, thus giving the diet its name.

Can this be true? It sounds kind of like magic or voodoo, right? In this book, we will explain the science behind the Keto diet, dispel the many myths and dangers associated with it and guide you through the process of choosing the correct kinds of food (and avoiding the others) that will turn your body into a fat-burning machine

What is This Book About?

In short, it's a guide, practical and scientific, that will help you decide if the Ketogenic diet is right for you and, if so, ease its integration into your life.

That's not all -- you will be treated to a multitude of delicious recipes that will help you to begin your weight-loss journey. Who said that you can't eat yummy stuff while losing weight? This book includes two weeks' worth of mouth-watering meal plans, recipes and shopping lists that will ease your transition to a healthy lifestyle.

When you're feeding your body the wrong things, your body will let you know. You'll get sick, have scarce energy and life will seem dull. With this book, you will learn how to fine-tune your food consumption for optimal health.

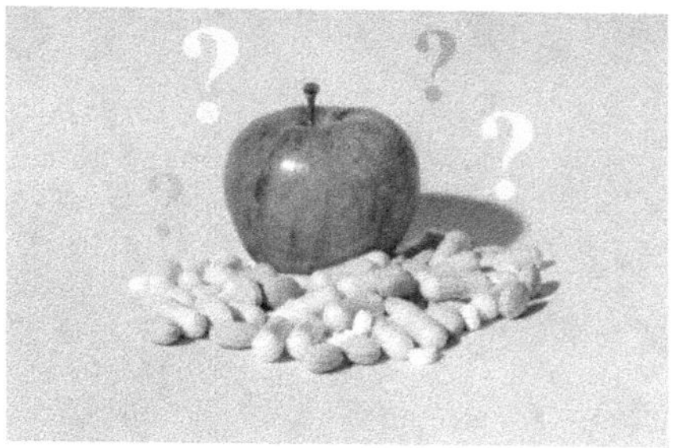

Listen to Your Doctor

Although I'll be giving you a lot of key information about keto, at the end of the day, nothing can replace the advice of your doctor.I encourage you to visit with your healthcare professional to discuss the changes that you will be making in your diet. He or she will answer your questions and probably encourage you to follow a diet that was pioneered successfully almost one hundred years ago.

Let Me Guide You Through It

I'm a living testimonial that keto works. It is because I have changed my lifestyle and followed the diet, that I know exactly what you need to learn and do to have the same (or better) success I've had.

In short, these are the things you'll need to learn, all of which I cover in this book:

- The proper steps to follow for starting the diet
- Permanent weight-loss strategies
- How to "ease" into the diet
- The dos and don'ts; what you can and can't eat/drink
- Meal plans, shopping lists, support, and **lots of keto-licious recipes.**
- Keto tips, tricks and hacks
- Techniques for sustainable keto
- Case studies and testimonials

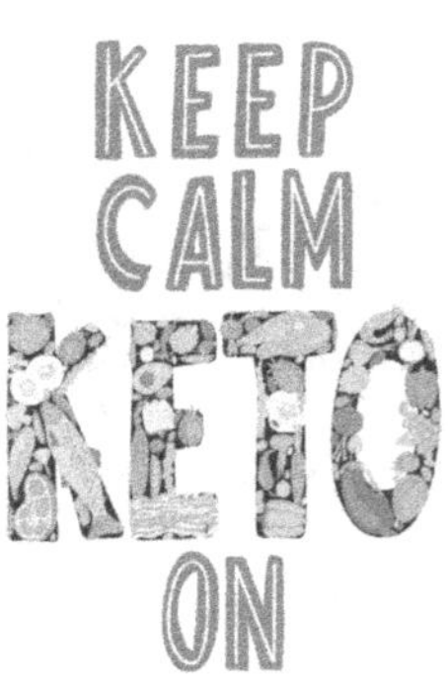

It is my sincere hope that this book helps to be the catalyst that begins your journey of weight loss and good health. I have walked in your shoes and know firsthand that it won't be easy. However, it will be worth it. You owe it to yourself!

PART I

INTRODUCTION TO THE KETO DIET

THE CASE FOR THE KETO DIET

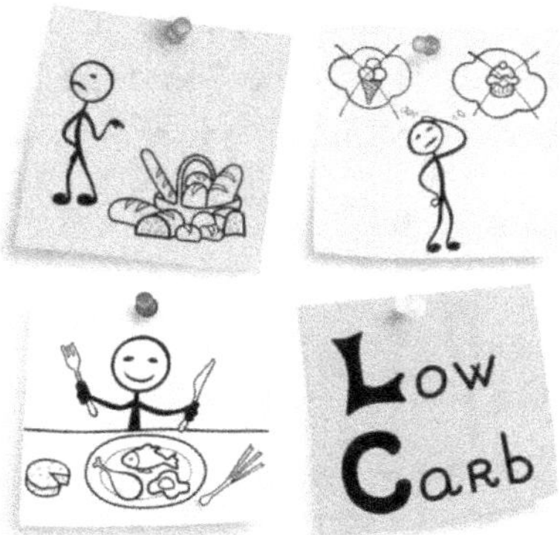

UNDERSTANDING THE KETO DIET

The Internet is filled with all kinds of information about the Keto diet. All this information can be somewhat overwhelming.As a result, I've decided to present to you a concise and easy way to understand the basics about the Keto diet.

The best way to understand the Keto diet is to understand that it is possible to change the way that your body gets its energy. With a carbohydrate-rich diet, your body is prone to convert carbohydrates into energy and never go near your fat reserves. By limiting carbohydrates to 20-25g net carbs a day and supplying your body with ample fat and protein, you can make it easier for your body to burn fat instead of glucose. Remember that the Ketogenic formula is 70% healthy fats, 20% protein and 5% carbohydrates.

Following this formula has many health benefits such as weight loss, enhanced energy and better blood sugar control. Subsequently, nourishing your body with a diet of healthy fats, proteins and very little carbohydrates, you will experience less hunger, even though you are consuming less calories. When you don't feel like you are starving yourself, you are more apt to maintain the Keto diet.

By choosing to follow this formula, you will boost your body into ketosisThe metabolic process of ketosis is when your body does not have enough glucose for energy. Without enough glucose, the body will turn to burning stored fats instead. The burning of stored fats causes a build-up of acids or "ketones" that the body uses for energy. So, a Ketogenic diet is a food plan that promotes the production of ketones.

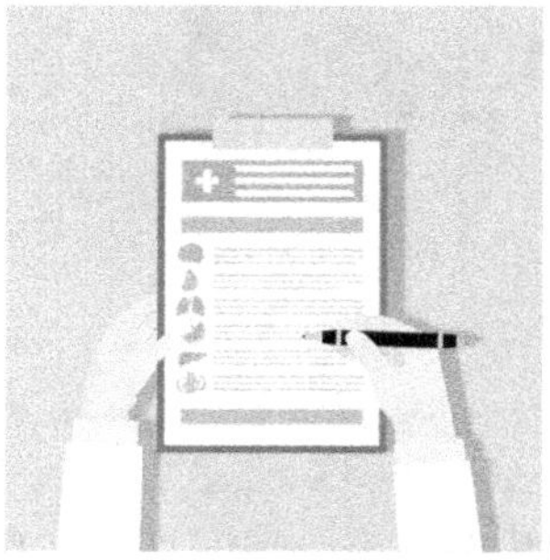

Low Carb, High Fat

In the 80s we feared fat. We learned that there were good fats, not so good fats and fats that would kill you. Foods like butter were banned from our diets. Heavy foods rich in dairy and fat were quickly replaced with low-fat items that were thought to be healthier for you.

This form of thinking was based on the fear that natural fat raised cholesterol which in turn put us at risk of health calamities like heart attacks.

In the latter decades of the 20th century we believed that high cholesterol was totally bad for us, when the truth was more complicated than that. There is good protective HDL A cholesterol and dense LDL particles that are not protective at all. In fact, when we don't have enough of protective HDL, bad things happen. For example, a low-fat diet can promote heart disease. Unbelievable, huh?

In a study published in the New England Journal of Medicine, the results were clear: people on a low-fat diet were more prone to heart disease. Further, another study found that people on a low-fat diet, had a higher incidence of diabetes. Even though these low-carb diets emphasized healthy carbs like fruit and fruit juice, more sugar found its way into these diets via refined products like pasta and white rice.

Bad Fat vs. Good Fat

Into the new century, people started searching for better results in their weight-loss and healthier eating. Foods like butter and eggs started making an appearance on weight-loss diets. Why?

The difference that changed the world of weight loss was better information and the widening definition of fat. No longer is there just bad fat but instead there are four categories: Saturated fats, monounsaturated fats, polyunsaturated fats and trans fats. Of these, trans fat is the worst villain.

Hydrogenation is the reason that trans fats are bad for you. Hydrogenation is a process where healthy oils are made into solids so that they will not spoil or turn rancid. This happens in a process that adds hydrogen atoms to the carbon chain turning oils into solids. A good example of this process is when vegetable oil is hydrogenated to make margarine. Foods such as fried foods, creamer, potato chips, doughnuts and frosted desserts all have hydrogenated ingredients in common i.e. hydrogenated oil.

· · ·

The Fat Villain

Saturated fats like those found in fatty beef, beef tallow (fat), lard and chicken with skin are the villains of a healthy diet. These foods are clearly not good for you and should be avoided.However, there is such a thing as a good saturated fat. The American Heart Association says that butter, cheese and red meats are fine if they are a limited part of your diet. Also, you can replace some saturated fats with healthier saturated fats. Such as replacing shortening or lard with coconut oil.

The fats that you will see a lot in a Ketogenic diet are monounsaturated fats and polyunsaturated fats. Polyunsaturated fats are found in foods that have Omega 3 and Omega 6 fats. The omega fats help reduce inflammation, keep healthy hormone levels and cell membranes. Omega 6 fatty acids do promote some inflammation in the body, but they protect and support healthy brain and muscle functions.

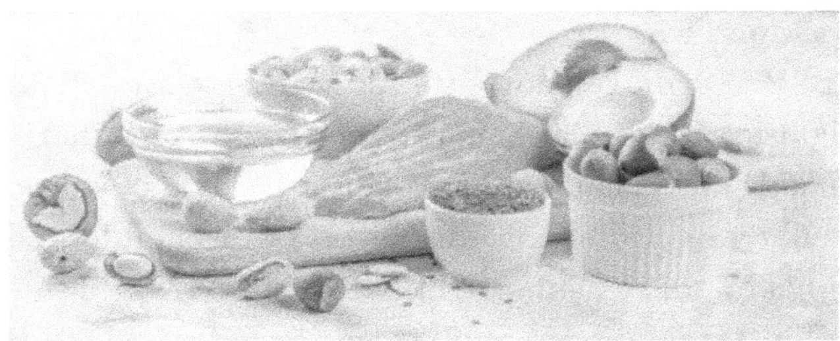

The Fats That Are Good for You

Other fats that are good for you are foods that have polyunsaturated fats such as fish (salmon, mackerel, herring, albacore tuna and trout) sunflower seeds, flax, soybean oil and safflower oil. However, not all polyunsaturated fats are good for you. Consuming products with soy and corn oil has been linked to a surge in body fat and inflammation.

Monounsaturated fats are not completely bad or completely good for you. Foods such as Avocados, macadamia nuts and olives (olive oils) aid insulin sensitivity, fat storage, weight loss and boost energy levels. Monounsaturated oils have also been found to look after the heart.

Monounsaturated fat-containing food to avoid are canola oil and peanuts, to name a few. In fact, the Ketogenic diet encourages the consumption of nuts except for peanuts as they are a legume that is high in carbohydrates.

Making Good Choices

The Ketogenic diet is one of many diets that promote the low consumption of carbs. Yet this does not mean that you must cut carbs completely out of your life. It's all about making good choices. For example, fruits like strawberries and blueberries will be a better choice than a banana or an apple. Bread made with almond flour is going to be a better choice than bread made with white flour. The Keto diet is all about making good choices.

Remember, the reason for low carbs is that you are trying to produce ketones that you will burn for energy. Too many sugars and processed food high in carbs may give you energy but in the long run it can make you feel bad. Insulin aids your body in turning glucose (sugar) into energy. When there is too much insulin, you can develop a situation where your body becomes resistant to insulin.

Busting Common Keto Diet MYTHS

Launching a diet that is unlike the familiar low-fat diet or even a typical low-carb diet comes with its share of truths and myths. Friends and family will have heard rumors that the Keto diet is unsafe or just a fad. Let's take the time to examine the modern myths and do some myth-busting.

Ketosis is Bad for Your Brain

As it happens, the brain runs on the energy provided by glucose. The Keto diet promotes the production of less glucose. In fact, the brain can run on the glucose produced from protein. Specifically, through the process of gluconeogenesis, the body can make glucose from dietary protein; so, it is not necessary to eat a high amount of carbs to produce glucose for the brain.

Following The Keto Diet Will Result in a Deficiency of Nutrients Delivered to Your Body

When people think of diets, they think of "less" and starvation. The Keto diet is about adding more fat and protein to your diet. Sure, you are eating less carbs but if you follow the Keto diet correctly, you will find that it adds nutrients, instead of taking them away.

Making Your Body Produce Ketones Makes You Develop The Dangerous Condition of Ketoacidosis

Ketoacidosis is a life-threatening complication of diabetes that happens when your body no longer makes enough insulin to break down fat as fuel. Ketoacidosis primarily happens in the late stages of diabetes. It is impossible for a person who produces even a small amount of insulin to go into ketoacidosis.

Ketosis Can Cause a State of Dehydration That Can Kill You Due to an Electrolyte Deficiency

When you are following the Keto diet, you will lose water and electrolytes; however, by drinking a healthy amount of water and consuming foods that are rich in sodium, potassium and magnesium (electrolytes) you will make up for the deficiency.

The Keto Diet Increases Your Chance of Heart Disease by Raising Your Cholesterol Level

The Keto diet promotes foods that are heart healthy. Furthermore, the belief that high cholesterol causes heart disease has been debunked. We now know that there is such a thing as a healthy cholesterol level.

The Keto Diet Causes Kidney Stones and Damages Your Kidneys

This myth comes from the fact that people think a Keto diet is all about large amounts of protein in your diet. Specifically, the misunderstanding is that you replace carbs with protein and basically eat nothing but protein. The reality is that the Keto diet puts a limit on the amount of protein that you caneat. Also, you do not eliminate carbs entirely. Moreover, it has not been found that high levels of protein causes kidney stones or damages your kidneys.

Good Things Happen on The Keto diet?

The Keto diet places the body in a state of ketosis that results in the production ofketones.Primarily, the Keto diet changes the fuel that your body uses for energy. When you eat a lot of carbs, your body has no interest in breaking down the fat in your body or even the fat in your diet. Carbs are converted into galactose, fructose and glucose. The body then uses glucose as energy because it has it in abundance, Conversely, when you eat a diet low in carbs, your body begins to use fat released from cells to produce ketones, which turn protein into glucose

Studies have shown that a diet of refined carbs and sugar produces high levels of glucose that can overwhelm the neural pathways with free radicals - toxic molecules - and glucose that can deplete antioxidants. This leads to an excess of oxidation and inflammation in the brain.

When a diet excludes or diminishes the ingestion of high amounts of carbohydrates, promoting the production of ketones, less free radicals are produced. Consequently, natural antioxidants easily "neutralize" free radicals. In this way, antioxidants are not depleted.

This information is new and still being tested by psychiatrists such as Dr. Georgia Ede. But it is an interesting medical study that shows how our mental health is tied to good nutrition.

The Keto diet was primarily developed to treat pediatric epilepsy, but since the 1920s, other health benefits have been found. Here is a list of them:

List of Benefits of The Keto Diet

- **Heart disease** - Taking away or lessening risk factors such as high body fat, HDL levels, high blood pressure and high blood sugar.
- **Cancer** - Keto diet has shown to have an impact on tumors.
- **Alzheimer's** - There is research to determine if the Keto diet can slow down progression and reduce symptoms.
- **Parkinson's disease** - Improves symptoms.
- **Polycystic ovary syndrome** - High insulin levels have been linked to POS.The Keto diet lowers insulin levels.
- **Acne** - Reduces the consumption of sugar and processed foods that can increase or cause acne.

The Keto Diet Case Studies

For over a hundred years, the Ketogenic Diet has been under examination by the medical community. In this chapter, we will examine some of the medical case studies that have tested and explored the benefits of the Keto diet.

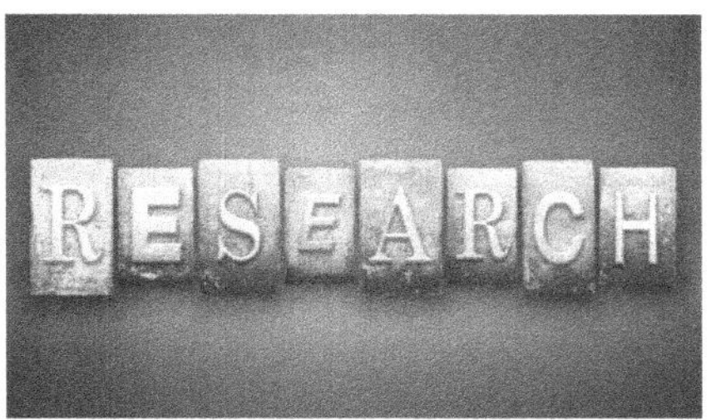

Very-Low Carbohydrate Ketogenic Diet v. Low-Fat Diet for Long Term Weight Loss. *British Journal of Nutrition (1)*

In this case study, researchers analyzed the results of several studies to find out which diet was more successful amongst patients who were engaged in weight loss. Specifically, the researchers were looking for the results of the Keto diet versus low-fat diets.

The researchers pored over each study and paid attention not only to the amount of weight lost but also the health of everyone that followed these diets. The researchers also paid attention to how long the patients stuck to these diets. The theory was that the longer the patient stayed on the diet, the more successful they would be at losing weight. Furthermore, the researchers wanted to know which diet was easier for the patients to follow: the low-fat diet or the low-carb diet?

After carefully studying all the different studies, the researchers discovered that overall, the patients who followed the Ketogenic diet lost more weight. Also, the researchers found that low-carb diets led to significantly favorable changes in body weight and the reduction of major cardiovascular risk factors. The conclusion of this case study was that following a low-carb diet such as the Ketogenic diet resulted in patients achieving a long-term decline in body weight and diastolic blood pressure.

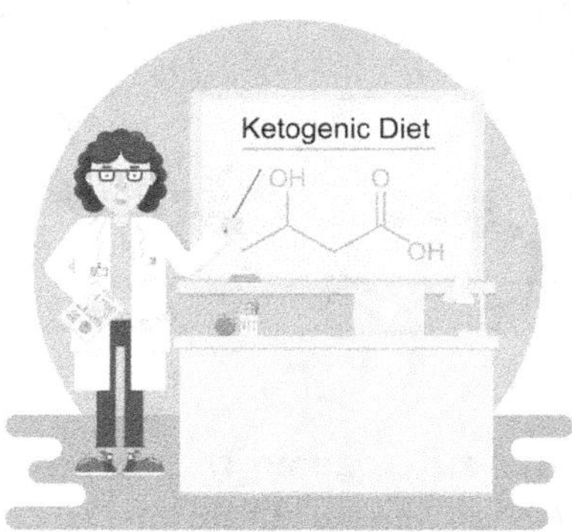

High-Protein Diets for Appetite Control and Weight Loss – The 'Holy Grail' of Dieting?*British Journal of Nutrition* (2009). (2)

For any diet to be effective, you've got to stay on it. Not only that, but the success of any diet depends on whether you feel full after you eat. If you feel that you are starving yourself, staying on the diet is going to be difficult. So the test is which diet will make you feel more full.

In this study, patients were required to eat 15% to 30% more protein in their diet. The test was to determine if the patients felt less hungry eating more carbs. The Keto diet fit the requirements of this study as the formula for it is: Fats 75%, Protein 20% and 5% carbs. So, you eat more protein than you do carbs.

The conclusion of this study was that indeed protein helps you feel satiated and therefore, you are more likely to stay on the Keto diet. And, the longer you stay on the diet, the more weight you are going to lose. Could the Keto diet be the holy grail of dieting?These researchers felt it was.

Reducing Diets: Weight Loss of Obese Patients on Diets of Different Composition. *British Journal of Nutrition (3)*

Two popular diets are the low-fat diet and the low-carb diet. In this study, patients were put on one of these diets and diligently observed. Researchers monitored the weight loss of each group for weight loss and the speed in which they lost that weight.

At the end of the study, it was concluded that patients on a low-fat high-carbohydrate diet had a slower weight loss and that they even gained some weight. However, the patients that were on a high-fat and high-protein diet lost weight faster at the beginning of the diet. In the end, all the patients lost weight no matter what diet they were on.

However, the researchers cautioned that individual choice and the palatability of the diet really made a difference. If you choose a diet that doesn't really have the food you like to eat, you might not stay on the diet and lose a good amount of weight. Yet, if you choose a diet with your favorite foods or foods you will eventually learn to enjoy, you will lose the weight in a healthy and happy way.

Dietary Protein – Its Role in Satiety, Energetics, Weight loss and Health. *British Journal of Nutrition, 108 (4)*

This study found that the Keto diet, with its low-carb features helped people to feel full and energetic even though they were limiting what they were eating. Increasing the amount of protein and decreasing the amount of carbs was key in feeling energetic and healthy. Patients who felt good while they were on a diet, stuck to the diet longer and lost more weight.

This study also found that there was no damage in the livers of patients who followed this type of diet.

Ketogenic Diet Benefits Body Composition and Well-being But Not Performance in a Pilot Case Study of New Zealand Endurance Athletes. *Journal of The International Society of Sports (5)*

In this study, researchers observed athletes on a Ketogenic diet.Of specific importance were the athlete's body composition and performance outcomes over a period of 10 weeks. The question was whether the Keto diet could provide the high-level energy that an athlete needs.

The result was that the athletes were able to maintain their peak exercise intensity following the Keto diet. At first, the athletes experienced lower levels of energy during exercise but as the diet progressed, the athletes found that they felt a lot better and recovered easier from their intense exercises. In the end, the athletes wanted to utilize a Keto diet because of the health benefits that they experienced.

Scientists Explain What We Do and Don't Know, *Vicky Stein Ethan Weiss, MD, and Raymond Swanson, MD, UC San Francisco edu-news (6)*

Doctors Weiss and Swanson who were conducting this study, found that "cutting back on carbohydrates has many metabolic benefits". The doctors concluded that the body processes a limited amount of carbs a lot more efficiently and with less insulin.

Doctor Weiss tried the diet himself for six months and found that he felt healthier and that his borderline pre-diabetes condition was cured. Both doctors concluded that the diet isn't dangerous, but they urge people who are at risk and taking medications for conditions like diabetes and high blood pressure, seek nutrition counseling and talk to their doctor prior to starting the Keto diet.In particular, the Keto diet is so effective, the body changes and the need for certain medications changes.

Long-Term Effects of a Ketogenic Diet in Obese Patients. *Experimental and Clinical Cardiology, Dashti, H. M., et al. (7)*

This study found that the long-term benefits of a Keto diet significantly reduced body weight of the patients in the study. Also, there was a decreased level of triglycerides, LDL cholesterol and blood glucose and increased level of HDL cholesterol. There were no significant side effects. Doctors concluded that it was safe to follow a Ketogenic diet long-term.

Extended Ketogenic Diet and Physical Training Intervention in Military Personnel, *Military Medicine, LaFountain et al.(8)*

Although many in the armed services are very active, there are some soldiers who have a problem with maintaining the required weight as designated by the military. The concern for these soldiers is that they be able to lose weight and keep the ability to perform at peak physical condition.

In this study, scientists wanted to know whether following a Ketogenic diet would help soldiers with the task of physical readiness and being fit. Obesity is a challenge for some soldiers so doctors wanted to know if the Keto diet could help. Scientists monitored military personal by observing their ketone production and with that data, personalized the soldier's Keto diet.

At the conclusion of this study, scientists found that the soldiers stayed on the diet and followed the Keto diet requirements without fail. Consequently, the soldiers lost weight and showed improvements in their body composition by losing visceral fat. Following the Keto diet did not compromise the soldiers' ability to perform physically.

Scientist found that the Keto diet was a "credible strategy to enhance overall health and readiness". At the end of this study, scientists concluded that soldiers could benefit from losing weight and improving their body composition with the Keto diet.

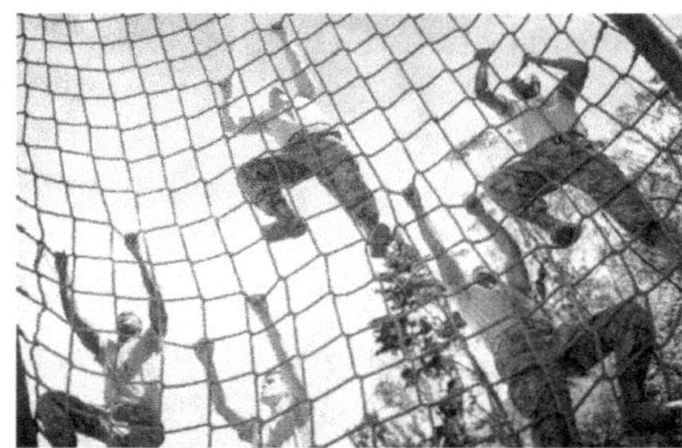

Ketogenic Diet. *[Updated 2019 Mar 21]. Masood W, Uppaluri KR. Stat-Pearls Publishing (9)*

In this book about the Keto diet, the researchers found that the Keto diet was not only an effective weight-loss plan but that the Keto diet also had health benefits such as improved blood pressure, blood glucose regulation and better cholesterol levels. The Keto diet also showed promising results with many different neurological disorders such as epilepsy, dementia, traumatic brain injury, acne cancers and metabolic disorders.

This study also found that the quality of calories consumed affected the number of calories that were burned. They also found that the Keto diet had a more significant impact on weight-loss compared to low fat diets.

Successful Treatment of a Patient with Obesity, Type 2 diabetes and Hypertension with The Paleolithic Ketogenic diet, *Csaba Tóth, Zsófia Clemens (10)*

Can following the Keto diet help patients become healthier? In this article, the researchers tracked the progress of a patient with metabolic syndrome who was heavily medicated. At the conclusion of this study, the patient was able to lose weight, discontinue her medication and improve blood glucose levels. Over the course of 22 months, she stayed on the diet and remained healthy as proven by blood tests. In conclusion, the researchers felt that the Keto diet was "feasible and cost-effective"

· · ·

Chapter Summary

- The Keto diet was developed almost one hundred years ago
- 75% Fat, 20% Protein, and 5% is the key formula to the Keto diet
- Not all fats are harmful
- There are many medical case studies that support the Ketogenic Diet

In the next chapter you will learn how to begin following the Keto diet.

2

—————

GROUND RULES

WELCOME TO THE WORLD OF THE KETO DIET. IN THIS CHAPTER YOU will learn what to add to your food plan and what to avoid. You will learn about getting your body into ketosis and how to measure ketosis. Further, you will learn about exercising while your body is in ketosis and ways to maintain ketosis in the long term. At first, when I started the diet, I found all this information to be overwhelming, so I have broken it down into easy-read info-bites for you. What follows is important and hopefully easy to understand.

Step 1: Food to Eat and Food to Avoid

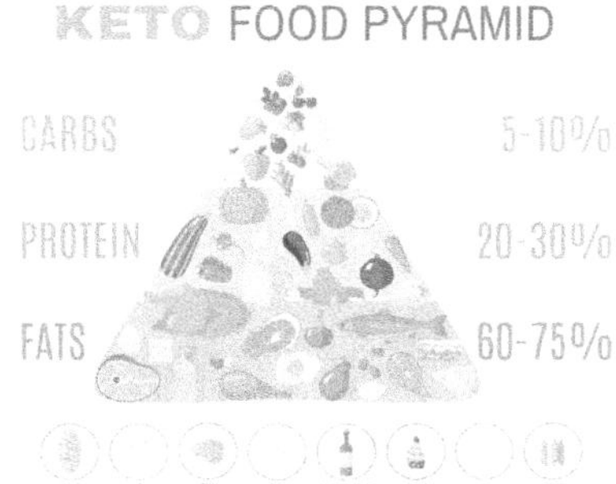

Food Pyramid According to Recommended Intake

Imagine a food pyramid with the keto foods that you are going to be planning your meal from. At the top will be berries, nuts and then dairy. These foods are to be eaten in a small amount. Then, for the middle of the food pyramid, you have non-starchy vegetables and protein.These foods should be the main components of your meals. And then on the bottom, where everything rests upon, you have healthy fats. This is the largest part of the food pyramid.

The Foods to Add to Your Meal Plan

Most diets are about what you can and cannot eat. Some diets even assign points to the food you eat; others emphasize counting calories. The Keto diet is all about getting your body to start burning fats instead of sugars that are produced when you eat carbohydrates.

The Following Are Foods That You Can Explore and Choose to Add to Your Diet:

Seafood

- Salmon
- Tuna
- Sardines
- Mackerel

- Trout
- Shellfish

Poultry

- Eggs
- Duck
- Chicken
- Turkey
- Quail

Meats

- New York Strips Steaks
- Ribeye Steak
- Pork Belly
- Lamb Chops
- T-Bone Steak
- Porterhouse Steak
- Baby Back Ribs

Dairy

- Greek Yogurt
- Hard Cheeses
- Soft Cheeses
- Cottage Cheese
- Sour Cream
- Whipping Cream
- Heavy Cream
- Cream cheese
- Butter

Vegetables

- Avocado
- Pumpkin
- Asparagus
- Zucchini
- Eggplant
- Spinach
- Kale
- Arugula
- Cauliflower
- Mushrooms
- Squash
- Broccoli
- Bell Peppers
- Cabbage
- Celery
- All varieties of lettuce

Fruits

- Raspberries
- Black Berries
- Blueberries
- Plums
- Strawberries
- Limes
- Lemon

Oils, Butters, Nuts and Seeds

- Avocado Oil
- Olives and cold pressed olive oil
- Flax Seeds
- Nuts
- Hemp Hearts
- Coconuts and unrefined coconut oil

- Nut and seed butters
- Chia seeds
- Cacao nibs

Miscellaneous Food

- Shiritaki Noodles
- Unsweetened coffee or tea
- Dark Chocolate
- Cocoa Powder

Foods to Avoid

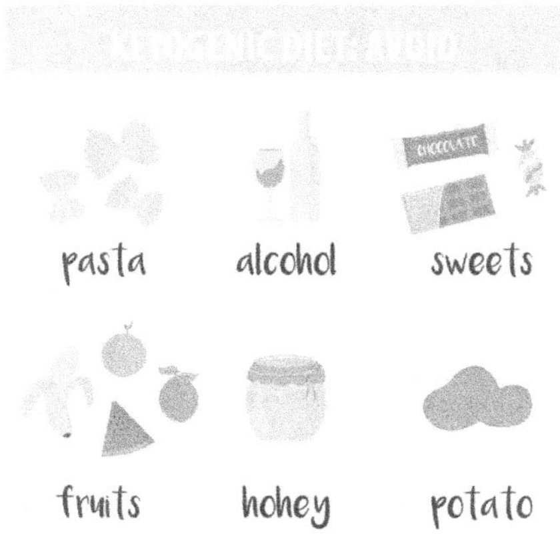

In the Keto diet, you will choose your carbohydrates wisely but there will be foods to avoid such as:

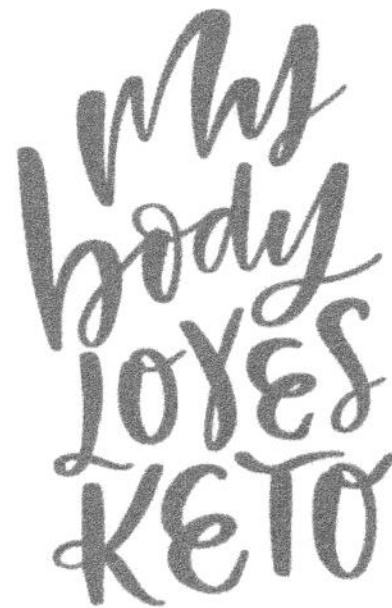

- **Grains and grain-based food:** wheat, corn, rice, pasta, granola, cereal.
- **Sugar and sugar sweetened products:** table sugar, soda, sports drinks, honey, agave, maple syrup.
- **Fruits that are high in sugar:** apples, bananas, oranges (Sometimes these fruits are allowed before exercising as they may encourage an energy boost).
- **Tubers and tuber-based food:** potatoes, potato chips, french fries, yams.
- **Alcohol**
- **Hydrogenated Fats**
- **Fast Foods**

The Dos and Don'ts of Alcohol

Pure alcohol does not have carbs and there are some alcoholic drinks that are very low in carbs. The alcohols that don't have carbs are: whiskey, tequila, gin, vodka and rum. Light beer and wine are also low in carbs. Pay attention to the mixers because they can be high in carbs. Avoid juice, soda and energy drinks. Mixers that have low carbs are: sugar-free tonic water, powdered flavor packets, seltzer and diet soda.

Alcohol can be a hard category to regulate but it is possible to plan ahead and fit alcohol into your Keto diet.Remember that mixed drinks can have added carbs. Examples are: regular beer, cosmopolitans, margaritas, whisky sours, bloody marys, sangrias and pina coladas.

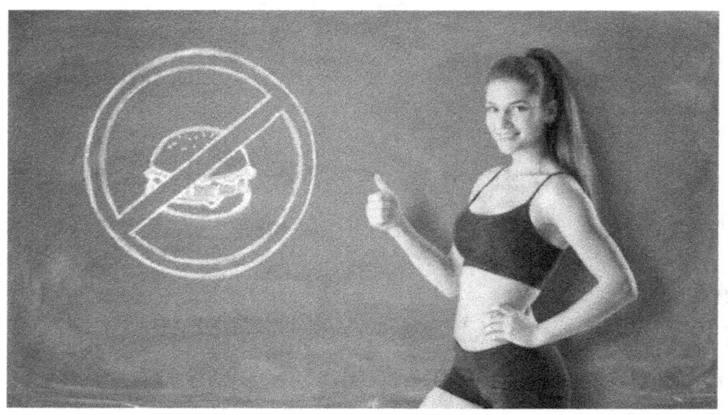

Fast food is Part of Our Culture But Should Be Avoided

Fast food, although very convenient, needs to be something that you learn to do without.In the meal planning section of this book, we will teach you which wholesome foods you can substitute for fast food. And of course, there is always a situation where you need to eat out. It is possible to find items on the menu that you can eat, and not throw off your meal plans. It's just that foods like french fries and fried chicken are not part of a healthy diet. Consequently, these foods need to be cut out of your diet. Fast food is part of our culture, but it is possible to learn other healthy habits that can satisfy your need for speed.

Categorizing Fruit in a Unique Way

While on the Keto diet, you will learn to think and categorize fruit in a new way. The glycemic index is a ranking of foods according to how they affect your blood glucose level. The traditional fruits that we are used to liking, oranges, apples and bananas are high in natural sugars. These fruits can raise your blood sugar as they are high on the glycemic index. Learn to choose berries like strawberries and blueberries for your meals or snacks. These berries contain some fiber and that makes these fruits rank lower on the glycemic index.

Fresh is the best, so avoid canned fruits and fruit juices that contain a lot of artificial ingredients and hidden sugars. The same can be said of canned vegetables and vegetable juice. It is better to seek out organic sources over foods that are processed and canned.

Avoiding Diet Foods

Foods that are marketed as diet foods should also be avoided or consumed with great caution. Diet sodas and diet candy (low-carb candy) can contain artificial ingredients that are just not good for you. These types of food are often modified in a way that adds chemicals and other ingredients that are not good for the body.

For example, aspartame, a key ingredient in some diet sodas and other diet products, has been observed to trick the body into thinking it is processing sugar. Specifically, aspartame can trigger the production of insulin which can place your body in fat storage mode. Accordingly, there are studies that link diet sodas and artificial sweeteners, to type 2 diabetes.

Tips When Eating Out

Sometimes eating out cannot be avoided. Many social events are scheduled at restaurants.For example, every kind of celebration ranging from birthday parties to graduations, often take place outside the home. Moreover, from time to time, business meetings are slated to convene during lunch or dinner. It's impossible to imagine that you will not eat in these situations. Not participating at a lunch or dinner can sometimes be thought of as unfriendly or in worst-case scenarios - hostile. So, how do you incorporate your new healthy way of eating into these must-be-attended social events?

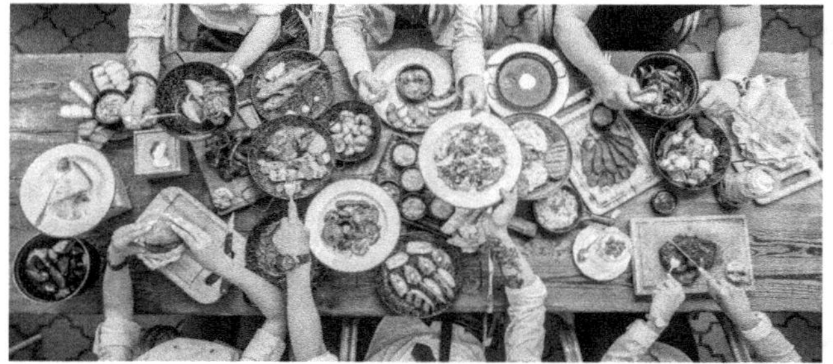

So often, it is not the specific food that needs to be avoided but the way it is presented. Healthy meats like turkey, cheese and chicken often come in the popular arrangement of sandwich or sub. Instead of ordering a sandwich or sub, request that your order become a salad or a power bowl. The contents of a sub or sandwich are almost always conducive to the Keto diet.Here are some examples:

- Turkey breast with provolone
- California club
- Chicken salad

When it comes to choosing a dressing for your requested salad, stick with olive oil and vinegar to avoid adding carbs to your meal.

Ask for Grilled Chicken Instead of Fried

Since the trend for eating healthy has begun, many restaurants now include a grilled option to replace fried foods. In fact, grilled chicken has become a premium item. Grilled chicken can be found in salads and power bowls. If grilled chicken is your entre, think about ordering a side of vegetables like green beans or coleslaw.

Iced Tea or Coffee Instead of Sodas

Although an acquired taste, teas served without sugar can be a delicious choice. Many restaurants are now brewing alternatives such as raspberry or peach tea that are tasty on their own without a sweetener.

Coffee is also another good choice and you don't have to skip the cream or milk. If you like almond or soy milk in your coffee, be sure that there is no added sugar.

A Different Kind of Burger Experience

Sometimes it is what you add to a burger and not what you take away, that contributes to a healthy eating experience. When eating out, I request a large lettuce leaf or two, to wrap my burger in. With all the tasty add-ons that are on your Keto diet meal plan, you won't mind not having a bun to contain your burger. Adding cheese, bacon, mustard, mayo, onions, tomatoes and guacamole to your burger can make you forget the bun that you aren't going to eat.

Power Bowls

Restaurants are now including food bowls on their menus. Many bowls include food ingredients that are straight off the Keto diet meal plan like: steak, eggs, tomatoes, avocado, spinach and bell peppers. What's more, these bowls are high in protein and high in taste. Join the power bowl revolution and choose a power bowl over traditional sandwiches or meals with rice as a base.

What About Wings?

Chicken wings in all flavors such as the famous Buffalo wings, are now a popular item on restaurant menus and can easily be added to a Keto diet. However, be careful of sauces like honey, barbecue or teriyaki and be sure your wings aren't breaded or battered.

Another bonus is that wings are usually served with blue cheese, ranch dressing, carrots and celery which are definitely on your Keto diet.

Breakfast for Lunch or Dinner

As eggs, sausage and bacon are staples of the Keto diet, you can never go wrong ordering these items. Sausage and bacon are processed meats and should be eaten less frequently.Nevertheless, when eating at a restaurant, these meats can be a better choice than other breakfast offerings, like pancakes.

Desserts and Other Treats

When it comes to desserts, we are used to eating highly sugared foods. Get creative and order a nice cup of sugar-free tea, iced or hot. A variety of cheeses and nuts can also be a treat. Think outside the box and order something that will be a treat and not bog you down with sugar.

To Sum Up, Do The Following When Eating Out:

- Plan ahead
- Cut out the starch
- Add healthy fats (like butter and olive oil)
- Choose drinks with care

Chapter Summary

Starting the Keto diet: First Key point

- There are foods that are on the Keto diet that you need to avoid

- There are many foods on the Keto diet that you can have
- Planning for success can help you when you eat out
- Be cautious about alcohol
- Avoid fast food

In the next chapter you will learn the next key point for Keto diet success.

3

THE HOW-TO

Identifying Individual Macros

I am not good at math, so I started to worry when I began reading about macronutrients.Just the name intimidated me. The reality of the situation is that once you get started paying attention to your macronutrients, it soon gets easier to understand them. Basically, you are paying attention to the fat, carbs and proteins in your diet. You are also paying attention to the gram count in each of your foods.

Many websites and apps are available to analyze what you are eating. Each "keto-calculator" will not only ask you about the food you are eating but other key factors such as: gender, age, height, weight, body fat percentage, activity level and deficit/surplus, (the number of calories you want to consume in order to gain or lose weight.)

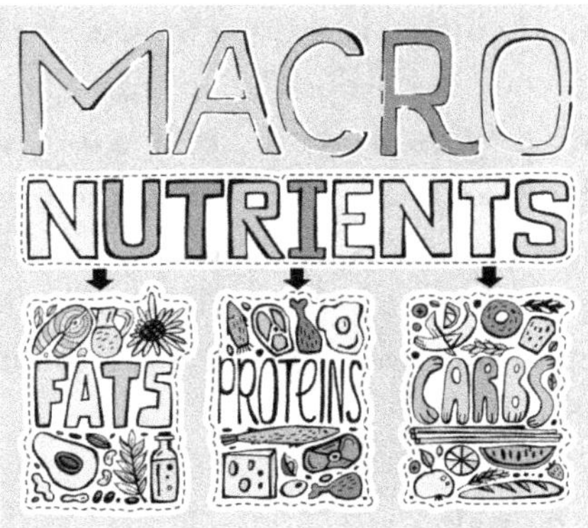

Calculating Your Macronutrient Ratio

A starting point in understanding what you need to eat, to reach ketosis, is to find out how many calories you need to eat daily. Although most diets aim at 2000 calories or less for weight loss, it is possible to customize those calories according to your personal statistics. The formula for figuring out the calorie numbers is called the Mifflin-St Jeor Formula.

The Mifflin-Jeor Formula in a Nutshell:

- **Men:** (10 x weight in kg) + (6.25 x height in cm) – (5 x age in years) + 5
- **Women:** (10 x weight in kg) + (6.25 x height in cm) – (5 x age in years)-161

Let's look at an example:
My weight is 90kg and I am 5 feet, 5 inches (165.1cm)
So, my Mifflin-Jeor Formula will look like this:
(10 x 90) + (6.25 x 165.1) - (5 x 54) - 161 = 1500.88 calories/day
My daily calorie intake will be: 1500

One size Does Not Fit All

Just as your calorie intake is unique to you, the same goes for the macronutrients of your Keto diet.For example, the suggested carb intake is 5% but you may need a bit more like 10%. It is perfectly okay to adjust your carb intake.The goal is to reach ketosis, not to adhere to a strict ratio of macronutrients.By watching for the signs of ketosis, you will know what percentage of carbs that you will need. Try a reasonable percentage for 2 weeks and then re-evaluate your needs.

An example of carb intake

Let us use the model of 1,500 calorie consumption for the day.To identify how many carbs, you need for your diet you can plug in this equation.Each gram of carbohydrate has 4 calories each.So the formula will look like this:

Let's stick to the model of 20% carbs for a 1500 calorie diet.

80 calories from carbs / 1,500 calories) x 100% = 5.3%

By dividing the number of total calories (carbs)by your total calorie intake (1,500) and then multiplying it by 100% you learn that you need to have 5.3 % carbs in your diet.

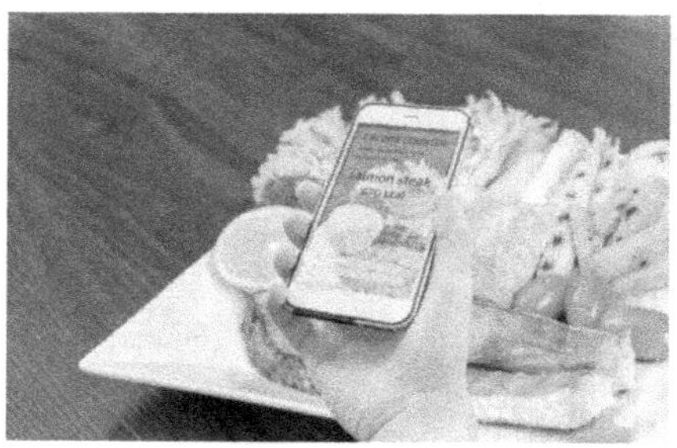

Counting Net Carbs

When it comes to counting carbs, you need to count the net grams not the whole total of carbs. At first, I had trouble with this until I learned this particular formula. When you eat a food that has a lot of fiber, you don't count the total numbers of carbs because the fiber is subtracted from the number as a whole

For example, one ounce of almonds has 11.9 total carbs and 9 grams of dietary fiber .The equation would look like this:

2 oz. of almonds have11.9 total carbs and 9 grams of fiber

11.9 - 9. = 2.9 net grams.

So, you would count 2.9 grams as net carbs

This is important to know because it reflects the way your body handles carbs.

What is Your Percentage of Fat Intake?

Fat has 9 calories per gram, so you need to calculate this with your calorie intake. A good place to start is 75% fat consumption. So, the equation will look like this:

1,448 x 75% ÷9 =121 grams

or 1,500 x 75% ÷9= 125 grams

So, this is the number of grams that you need, to insure the correct percentage of fat to add to your meal plan.

Protein for Your Body

If we use the above numbers of fat and carbs, we have 18% left for protein. To find out the number of grams, you multiply the number of calories by 18% and then divide by 4 (calories in each gram of protein)

The equation looks like this:

1448 x 18% ÷ 4 – 65

So you will need 65 grams to complete your macronutrient totals.

By The Numbers

Now that you have the equations, you have the tools to re-evaluate your diet every month. Knowing the most accurate amount of macronutrients that you need to consume will help you get to a state of ketosis. Another thing to consider is that although certain foods might be technically on the list of foods that you can have on the Keto diet, they might not fit into your macronutrient allowances.

I love ice cream and technically, if I find ice cream that does not have sugar, I am left with a food that is high in fat. Consequently, is this the right choice for me? Will I be getting the nutrients that I need for the day? No, I will not so I must look closely at the macronutrients I am including in my Keto diet that day.

Getting Physical

In chapter 3, I describe the different exercises that are ideal for a person on the Keto diet.Considering the type of energy that you will be expending, you will have to adjust the number of macronutrients; specifically, carbs, into your macronutrient equation. Use your discretion when adding carbs to your diet. Common sense and a bit of math, plus data, can help you in this endeavor.

Another thing to consider is the way you feel during and after your exercise. Match these feelings or body reactions to the signs of reaching ketosis, and you will have a clearer understanding of the macronutrients that you need to add to your diet.

Will My Brain Explode?

I am not great at math and numbers. In fact, sometimes, all these different equations make me feel like my head is going to blow up. If you have the same struggle, I suggest that you find apps and websites that will help you to find how many grams of fat, carbs and protein to eat on a daily basis – Keto diet calculators are an easy answer to your math dilemma.

To find these handy apps and websites, just use the following keywords:

- Keto calculator
- Keto macro calculator
- Macro calculator

- You can also search these terms with "free" in the key word phrase.

It is important that you find a calculator that is easy for you to use and available on the device that will be the most convenient for you. Sometimes I just pick a day of the week to sit down and work the numbers. Other times, I like to calculate my numbers daily.

Resources to Find the "Grams" in Food

I also keep a list of the grams of my favorite foods. As in this book, you can look at the nutrition information at the end of each recipe. You can also look at food nutrition labels on the package of the food you are preparing.

There are many carb gram charts on the internet. You can print one out or save it to the device that is most convenient to you.Keywords to search for these charts are as follows:

- The essential carb counter
- Carb counter calculator
- Protein calculator
- Fat calculator

Other types of apps or websites that are good to use as a resource are those that calculate the nutrition of any meal or recipe that you will be eating. Good keyword for this are:

- Food calculator
- Nutrition calculator
- Recipe nutrition calculator

Reach and Maintain Ketosis

The most amazing feeling is reaching ketosis and watching the pounds just melt away.Once you reach ketosis, it is important that you maintain it. There are going to be days that you have more energy than other days. By keeping and tracking information, you can adjust the Keto diet to suit your needs.

For example, I have mentioned carb loading before an intense exercise session. You might see that all you need is a piece of fruit to get that extra burst of energy. You might be tempted to eat bread or pasta – and if you do, record the amount of energy you get from those carbs and compare it to the day you just had some fruit. Did you get the same results?Did you have energy? Did you lose weight?

Tailoring Your Food Plan

The best thing about the Keto diet is that you can tailor it to fit your needs. In the following chapter, you will be presented with a two-week meal plan, recipes and a shopping list. With your daily journal and the meter of your choice: urine or blood tests (I will talk more about this later), you can learn what foods help you maintain a state of ketosis. Keto meal plans are not written in stone – they are meant to be revised and improved according to the results that you are experiencing. So, choose your testing method, gather information and enjoy tailoring your Keto diet to meet your needs.

Concentrate on Your Protein Intake

Preparing yourself for a Keto diet is very important. Planning is the key to success. Here are some steps that you can take to ensure your weight loss victory.

In the beginning, you need to be mindful of how you are going to switch from eating carbs and proteins. Too much protein can be hard on your kidneys, so it is important to hit the sweet spot of 20% high quality protein. This is a tremendous change for anyone that is used to a diet full of carbs. Thinking of how you can put more protein in your diet is key. Start making a mental list of good proteins that you love and think of ways that you can replace carbs with those proteins.

. . .

Personal Experience

When I started the Keto diet, I thought that eating any and all protein was part of the meal plan. I would eat hot dogs and processed meat with a lot of additives. Also, I misunderstood that low-carb meant no carb. Consequently, I began to feel ill because I did not have the special nutrients that only carbs can bring to a diet.

Learn to Understand How Fat Fits into The Keto diet

In a Keto diet, the amount of fat you eat is negotiable. Unlike proteins and carbs, the amount of fat you eat can differ according to your goals. It is important that you learn how much fat in your diet makes you satisfied and then limit your intake. Another important point is to learn how much fat to decrease in order to lose weight.

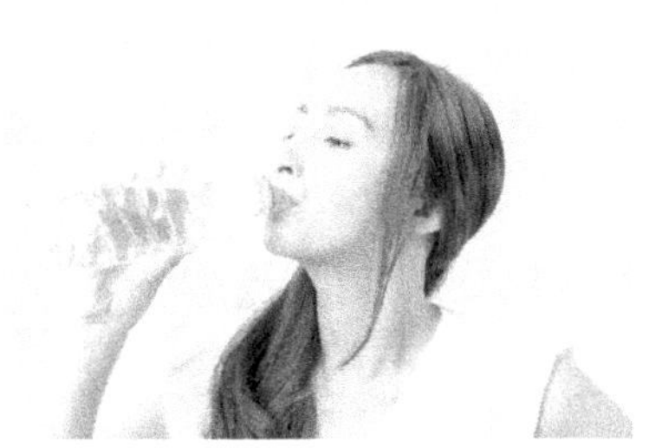

Increase Your Water Intake

The low-carb lifestyle requires that you drink more water. Specifically, it is good to aim not just for eight cups of water a day; but instead, aim higher and drink sixteen cups. It sounds like a lot but here is the reason for this increase: glycogen is stored in the liver where it binds to water molecules. When you eat less carbohydrates, this depletes the glycogen that is allowing you to burn fat. This also means that you are storing less water; and therefore, you might run the risk of becoming dehydrated if you do not add more water to your diet. So, to avoid becoming dehydrated, it is important to adopt the habit of drinking 16 cups of water a day.

Adding Crucial Electrolytes to Your Body

Since a low-carb diet decreases the amount of water you store in your body, you run the risk of flushing out crucial electrolytes such as sodium, potassium and magnesium. Losing these electrolytes may cause you to experience the "keto flu". However, there are ways to prevent this, mainly adding these electrolytes to your body. Eating foods such as bone broth, pickled vegetables and adding salt to your diet can help add these crucial electrolytes. Also taking supplements that contain these electrolytes can really help you. Before you start the Keto diet, it is good to keep in mind the foods that you will be adding to your meal plan that will keep you from feeling sick.

Learning to Eat Only When You Are Hungry

It is important to strengthen your resolve and stick to your meal plan. Following the Keto diet will help you to feel full when you eat your meals. Therefore, snacking or eating extra meals is not necessary anymore. Some of your off-plan eating can be due to your emotions such as stress or boredom. I always used to eat more when I was approaching a work deadline. It is beneficial to start a log of how you feel when you eat, so that you can identify the times that you are straying from your meal plans when you are not hungry. Doing this can help with your transition into the Keto diet.

Cutting Out Processed Foods

It is often easier to grab a hot dog or a ready-to-eat food that is considered to be a processed food. However, as you begin to plan your new Keto diet meals, become aware of the natural and whole foods that are just as easy to reach for. Start to study the new recipes in your meal plan so that you can easily learn innovative techniques for making food that is not processed. Eating whole or natural foods is a new way of finding sustenance and with a bit of preparation, including these foods in your diet, can be just as easy as the shortcuts you are taking with processed foods.

Increasing Your Activities Through Exercise

Adding exercise to your lifestyle can help you lose weight faster. With a healthier outlook, you will begin to feel better about yourself.- Following the Keto diet is going to give you a new lease of life and energize everything you do. Prepare to use that added energy in a way that will help you. Exercise is vital not only to weight loss but also to your emotional well-being. Preparing yourself to lead a more active life will be greatly beneficial to you.

Chapter Summary

In this chapter, I explained some of the steps you need to take to start a Keto diet:

- Step 1: Foods to eat and food to avoid
- Step 2 Identifying individual Macros
- Step 3: Getting into Ketosis Quickly
- Step 4: Testing your Ketones and making adjustments
- Step 5: Reaching and maintaining ketosis

Now that you know how to start the Keto diet, you have the keys to getting your body healthy. Are you ready? Are you excited?

Great! Let's move to the next chapter and learn some more key points for success.

4

FACTORS FOR SUCCESS

WHEN I WAS STARTING OUT ON THE KETO DIET, I FOUND SOME information about fasting that became a game changer for me. Starving yourself is the most primitive way to lose weight.You just don't eat. This is the case for many diets. However, there is a smart way to fast and still give your body the nutrients that it needs.This fasting is called intermittent and you will learn all about it in this chapter.

Getting into Ketosis Quickly

It is important to quickly get into ketosis when you are on the Keto diet because when you are in ketosis, the body converts fat into ketones and starts to use these ketones as your main source of energy. Getting into a state of ketosis requires a little bit more than cutting out carbs. It is essential to plan your meals and exercise so that you will be successful in putting your body into ketosis.

The State of Ketosis and Intermittent Fasting

Although I have been encouraging you not to go without food for an extended period, there are advantages to fasting for short periods of time.

The key factor to losing weight is to decrease the number of calories that you are taking in.Taking in too many calories at one time causes reactions in your body that encourage the storage of fat in the body. The relationship between the Keto diet and intermittent fasting is similar. In both states, intermittent fasting and ketosis, you are burning fat. The best time to fast is when you have achieved ketosis for a good amount of time. You will not experience a dramatic drop in insulin production; therefore, you will not have extreme reactions

The Basics of Fasting

Providing your body with more food than the body needs for energy, causes the pancreas to release more insulin. This insulin causes the body to store those extra calories for future use.The idea behind fasting is to produce the metabolic state of fasting – which of course is the opposite of the state of being fed.When cells are experiencing the state of fasting, they adapt and even become more resistant to diseases. In fact, as a response to fasting, your body gets stronger and finds better ways to function. This is the reason that scientists have concluded that fasting for short periods of time are beneficial to our bodies.

Different methods of fasting

Here are some methods of fasting that are popular:

- Restrict your eating window and then fast for no longer than 16 hours (The 16/8 intermittent fasting method)
- Eat normally for five days but only eat 500-600 calories for two days (5:2 diet)
- Fasting for 24 hours once or twice a week (Eat-Stop-Eat)
- Fasting every other day - only allowing 500 calories on fasting day (Alternate Day fasting)

- Eat a huge meal at night and only small amounts of raw fruits and vegetables during the day (The Warrior Diet)
- Occasionally, just skip a meal (Spontaneous Meal Skipping)

There Are Benefits to Intermittent Fasting

Intermittent fasting helps your body to avoid blood sugar spikes and low-grade inflammation. When you don't have this happening to you, your brain runs more efficiently, and you achieve mental clarity.

Intermittent fasting also helps to improve exercise performance. There's also evidence that a body running in tip top shape, can also reduce the risks of certain diseases such as cancer.Moreover, intermittent fasting has been found to increase your stamina.

Here is a List of The Benefits of Intermittent Fasting

- Reduces calorie intake
- Lowers insulin levels
- Stimulates fat burning
- Increases the rate at which the body burns fat in a resting state

Caution While Fasting

If you are a diabetic, you must check your blood glucose level and make medication adjustments. Talk with your doctor about fasting so that he or she can recommend proper ways to fast and not put yourself at risk.

It isn't wise to let yourself get dehydrated when fasting. Drink a lot of liquids while fasting.This doesn't count as breaking your fast – unless you have something high in carbohydrates like a soda.

Also, don't fast while you are pregnant.Depriving yourself of essential macronutrients can put you and your baby at risk.

. . .

Signs That You Need to Break Your Fast

If you begin to feel weak, shaky and your thinking is altered (having a brain fog), it is time to break your fast. There is such a fine line between the weight you lose when you are following the Keto diet and the weight you lose when you are fasting. Consequently, it is not necessary to torture yourself and fast for long periods of time. If you aren't able to fast without experiencing uncomfortable reactions/symptoms, don't worry about it. You will still be losing weight as long as you are in ketosis.

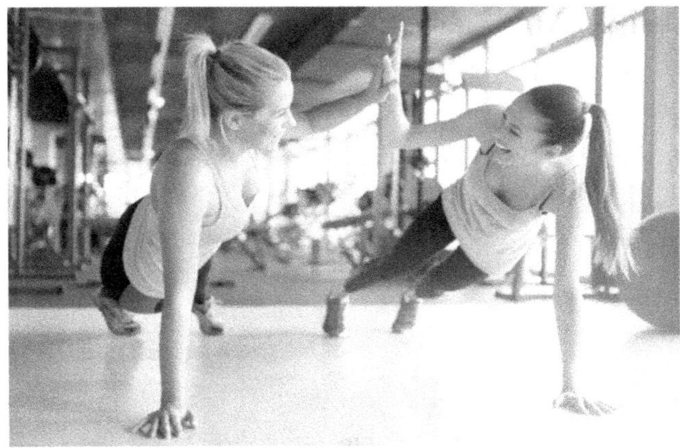

Consistency with Keto Diet and Exercise

Exercise is always part of a healthy diet plan and the Keto diet is no exception. Although the stress of exercise can kick you out of ketosis, your body will adjust over time and you will find that you can stay in ketosis as you exercise.

To help your performance when you exercise, you can raise your carbs to 25-60gms thirty minutes before you start exercising. This can be done by eating healthy carb foods like apples, oranges or bananas.

Both fat and glucose are used to fuel your muscles; moreover, if your glucose stores are very low, your body will use fat as your body's primary fuel. It is important that you pay attention to your body and its physiology. After an intense exercise session, when your insulin is on point, the number of ketones that are in your body may lower. If you feel this happening, add some MCTs (oil supplements) to your meal plan, so that your body can produce more ketones and replace what it lost. It is important to do this because MCTs cause your blood level of ketones to rise slowly over a period of time. Doing this will bring you back to the state of ketosis.

Exercises That Can Help

Many sources argue that exercise on the Keto diet is difficult. Specifically, intensive exercise pushes your body to its limits; making carbs essential for providing energy throughout the exercise. It is important to eat quality food on the Keto diet. The difference between eating hot dogs and steaks are immense.

In my experience, low intensity workouts are enough to keep me in shape and help me to sustain ketosis. Here are some examples:

Aerobic Exercise

- Cardio that lasts over 3 minutes
- Keto diet friendly as it burns fat.

Anaerobic Exercise

- Weightlifting for short durations and high intensity
- This exercise burns carbs.
- It is good to have some extra carbs, such as an apple or an orange, for a good burst of energy.

Flexibility Exercise

- Yoga, stretching
- Supports soft tissue and increases range of motion.

Stability Exercises

- Core training improves balance and supports body control and alignment.
- Helps regulate metabolism.

Low Intensity and Burning Body Fat

It is good to know that low intensity exercises use body **fat** as the key energy source; and, high intensity anaerobic exercise uses **carbs** as the foremost source of energy. Subsequently there may be a need to adjust your Keto diet to your exercise requirements.

The Keto diet is flexible, so it is possible to eat what you need, to produce the right fuel in your body. Simply eating a piece of fruit thirty minutes before you exercise can give you the energy for a high intensity workout like lifting weights. Concentrate on eating 15-30 grams of fast-acting carbs. An orange, for example, has 11 grams of carbohydrates and a banana has 27 grams.

Appropriate Amounts of Glycogen

The key to maintaining ketosis is to give your muscles the proper amount of glycogen.Raising the amount of carbs for exercise should not throw you out of ketosis. The idea of eating less and exercising more does not apply to the Keto diet. Paying attention to the quality of food that you eat is a lot more crucial than not eating. Choose meat, dairy and seafood that is of superior quality. I think of this as the hot dog versus steak argument, in my mind.

Also start gradually with low intensity exercises like bike riding or yoga. Keto cycling, which is taking a day or two to eat more carbs can also be part of your exercise plan. At the beginning you may feel sluggish and tired but the more you balance the carbs that you are eating, the better you will feel.

To sum up, follow these key points:

- Eat less carbs
- Including medium-chain triglycerides (MCTs) in your diet
- Become more physically active and begin an exercise program
- Step-up your fat intake with healthy fats
- Engage in a short or a fat fast
- Sustain a satisfactory protein intake
- Measure your ketone levels and fine-tune your diet as needed

The Keto Flu

The change that will happen to your body when you start the Keto diet affects people in different ways. One of the most common symptoms of change is the keto flu. The actual flu is a virus whereas the keto flu is more like your body is experiencing a withdrawal to something that is no longer plentiful – mainly carbohydrates. Instead of being singled out as a withdrawal, this reaction has been called the keto flu because the symptoms/reactions are similar to those that you get when you catch the actual flu.

The Symptoms of The Keto Flu

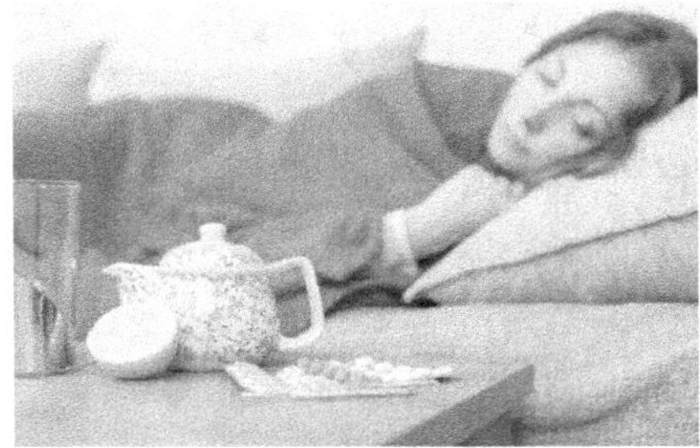

The onset of the keto flu means that you have brought your carbohydrate level of ingestion to a minimum, that there is an electrolyte imbalance and an altered hormone state. The basic symptoms are:

- Lack of mental clarity (brain fog)
- Diarrhea
- Fatigue
- Abdominal cramps
- Sleepiness
- Upset stomach
- Headaches

The Keto flu usually only lasts for a few days and at the longest two weeks.

How to "Treat" The Keto Flu

In some cases, a person is addicted to carbohydrates and will have a tough time introducing the body into a state where there are very little carbs entering their system. It is wise to gradually reduce carbs at first.

The first place to look to cut carbs is in foods that do not give you a lot of nutrients like sodas, pizza, pasta and potato chips. You can still snack and have fun with your food. You will just have to introduce new foods to your diet like coconut, cheese and avocados. Each of these foods is high in good fats. In fact, it would not be a bad thing to snack regularly in the beginning, even if you don't feel like eating. Simply eating small amounts of food more frequently, will help stabilize your blood sugars, which is very important in the initial phases of adapting to the Keto diet.

Schedule Your Changes

Here is a schedule I followed to prepare myself for the Keto diet:

- **Week 1** - Cut out all beverages with sugar
- **Week 2** - Cut out all sugary snacks
- **Week 3** - Cut out starchy carbs

When your body starts to rely on fat for energy instead of carbohydrates, you will experience many good changes in your body.

Chapter Summary

In this chapter, I explained some more basics about the Keto diet

- Intermittent fasting can help you reach your goals
- Steps to get into and maintain ketosis
- Healthy exercise that will help you achieve your goal
- All about the Keto flu and how to resolve it
- Tips to withdraw from eating a lot of carbs

There are a lot of ways to sustain your keto progress. In the next chapter, you will learn to use tools to measure your ketones.

5

MAKING PROGRESS

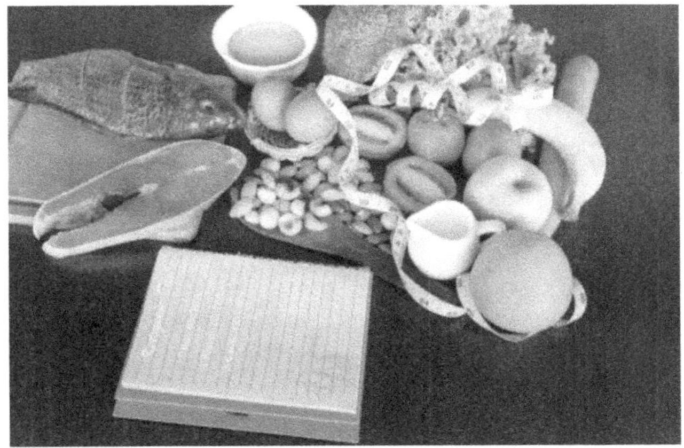

I have tried a lot of diets that just weren't for me. Sometimes the calorie count was too much for me and I didn't lose weight. Other times, I exercised and counted points and still I couldn't drop any pounds.

The Keto diet is very different. By testing and observing, you can tailor the Keto diet to work for you. As you have been learning, getting the body to use fat for energy is the goal of the Keto diet.

Knowing what level of protein and carb consumption gets your body to go into ketosis and stay, is important.

Not having glucose to burn as a power source, your body will begin to break down your fat reserves and make glycerol and fatty acids that turn into units called ketones. These ketones carry energy to the nervous system, brain and muscles. This process of switching over to burning ketones, preserves your lean muscle mass.

Monitoring your body for ketones

Measuring certain physiological conditions in your body is essential to knowing whether you are in ketosis or not. There are three ways to check for ketosis: keto strips that check ketones that are in your blood or urine, and a breathing apparatus that checks your breath for ketones.

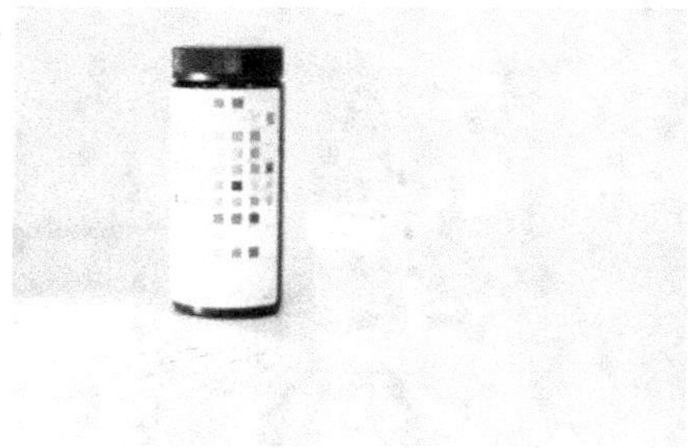

Keto Strips

Keto strips measure the ketone levels in your body. These strips are inexpensive and can be bought on Amazon or at your local CVS or drugstore. The keto strips measure whether you have two of the three types of ketones: acetoacetic acid and acetone.

Using the strips is a lot like testing the ph. level of water. You can either pee on the stick or use a container to catch your pee and then dip the strip in it. Almost at once, the strip will turn a certain color. Usually there is a chart on the strip container that will correspond with the color of your strip. Consequently, you will learn whether you have reached ketosis or not.

The time of day you take the test can make a difference. You might have more ketones in your system in the evening than you do in the morning or vice-a-versa. Sticking to the same time of day for your tests is the ideal way of checking your ketones.

Keto strips are good to use at the beginning of the diet. However, as your body gets more efficient at producing and using ketones, you will not be releasing as many ketones into your urine. Also, the strip only measures two out of three acids, so you need to keep that in mind for the validity of the results.

Keto Strip Testing Procedure

1. Wash your hands and then take a urine sample (in a container)
2. Immerse the right end of the keto strip into the sample for a few seconds
3. Wait the suggested time for the stick to change colors
4. Compare the strip with the chart on the package

Measuring Ketones with a Blood Strip

Another more reliable way to learn if you are in ketosis is the blood strip. You can buy a keto blood test monitor, or you can use a blood glucose meter that also reads the blood keto strips.These strips are a bit more expensive ($1 per strip) but they keep 12-18 months versus a urine strip that only lasts 6 months.

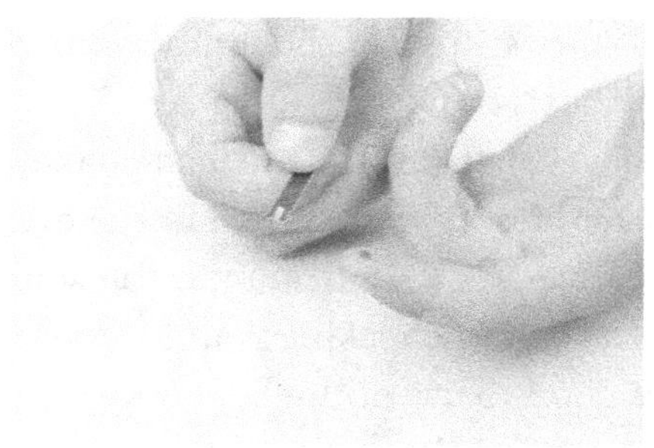

How to Use a Blood Strip:

1. Wash your hands
2. Place the lancet into the meter
3. Prick your finger with the lancet
4. Put a drop of blood onto the strip
5. Check the results
6. Dispose of the strip and the lancet
7. Refer to the box to compare your blood level of ketones for dietary ketosis.

Unlike the urine strip that measures acetoacetic acid and acetone, the keto blood meter test measures BHB – (beta-hydroxybutyrate) which is one of three types of ketones.

Testing for Breath Ketones

Purchasing a breath ketone meter to measure the number of acetones in your breath is another way to check the effectiveness of your Keto diet. At some point, you will notice that your breath smells fruity. This "fruitiness" is caused by the acetones in your breath. Measuring these acetones with a breath ketone meter can tell you whether you are in ketosis or not. Not as exact as blood or urine testing, the breath meter will tell you if you are in a general state of nutritional ketosis where your body is burning fat rather than glucose for fuel.

The difference with this meter is that once you put out the money to buy it, there are no strips to buy. The method of measuring ketones in your breath is accurate and non-invasive but keep in mind that it is not as precise as a blood test.

The Procedure of Testing Your Breath

1. Blow into your meter until the monitor flashes a green or red color
2. Notice how long the green or red-light flashes (green equals least acetone – red equals most acetone)
3. Count the number of times that the light flashes to indicate your ketone level

Using the breath meter can take a little longer than a urine or a blood test, as you must blow into the device until it can measure the acetone in your breath.

Testing your body to see if it has reached the state of ketosis can be done with urine or blood meters. The breath meter is less accurate but non-invasive and overall least expensive to use.By monitoring your ketones, you will be able to better tailor the Keto diet to your needs.

Keeping a Food Journal

Recording what you eat daily can become a routine that is quick and painless. Paying special attention to the amount of fat, protein and carbs that you are eating can make a big difference with the amount of success you can achieve on the Keto diet. Further, if you record your energy levels and the way that you feel, you will get a good impression of how the Keto diet is working for you. Specifically, observing these factors and tracking them daily are key to knowing if you have achieved ketosis. Taking the time to record your daily eating and how you feel can easily become part of your routine. I've designed some worksheets for your food journal in chapter 9.

I found that recording what I eat in my journal is a good indicator of my progress.It also reinforces the good choices that I am making. What kind of habits will you acquire, that will bring you to keto success?

Chapter Summary

- Keto diet Success is all about observing important factors in your body
- Checking for ketones in your urine is a good way to see if you have reached ketosis
- Checking for ketosis is a bit more efficient with a blood test
- Keeping a food journal or diary can help you analyze the facts

In the next chapter you will learn tips that will help you to stick to the Keto diet.

6

CONSISTENCY: DIET AND EXERCISE

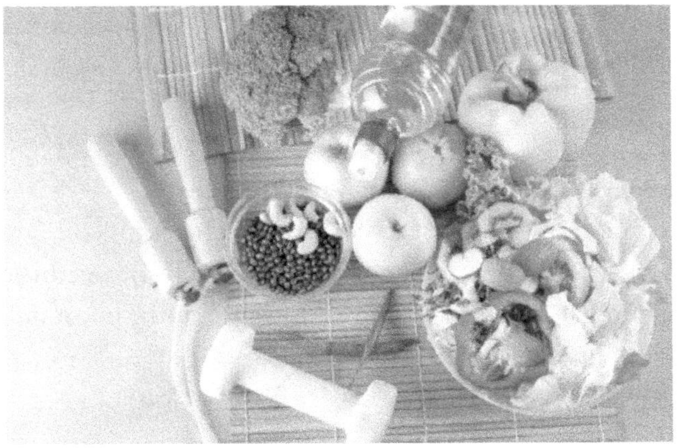

YOU HAVE BEEN LEARNING ABOUT HOW IN A DIET WITH A HIGH CARB intake, glucose is the primary source of fuel. However, you also learned that your body can use other fuel sources such as fatty acids and ketones or ketone bodies. This is the most important lesson of this book. Yet, how do you sustain the progress when you are on the Keto diet? I am not a machine and there were just some days that I couldn't keep up with my diet. Those were the days that I was in a kind of freefall. I don't want you to go through this same feeling, so I have written some key points and suggestions to help you stay consistent with your Keto diet.

Some of these key points are mentioned in the prior chapters but I share them in this chapter to emphasize their importance.

Amount of Carb Restriction

Although a common amount of carb limit is 20 grams, the amount can vary amongst individuals. Some people can eat as much as 40 grams and still get into a state of ketosis. In the beginning, your food plan will start with a low number of carbs and then you will work up from there, learning how many carbs you can consume and still maintain ketosis.

When you lower your carb intake to 20 grams or lower, your body levels of glycogen and insulin are reduced, causing fatty acids to be released from the fat stores in your body. The liver converts fatty acids into ketones. The body then uses these ketones as fuel.

Eat More MCTs (Medium Chain Triglycerides)

MCTs (medium chain triglycerides) like coconut oil, are quickly absorbed and turned into ketones by your liver. As little as one teaspoon a day at first, and then two to three tablespoon daily, over a week's time, can help you to get into ketosis.

Exercise

Taking part in physical activity can require your body to find more energy. If you have restricted your carb intake, your body will be using ketones for energy. The more energy you require from exercising, the more ketones you will need for fuel.

Good Fats

The consumption of good fats like olive oil, avocado oil, coconut oil, butter and lard, are low in carbs and can help you to reach ketosis. Choosing fats from different plant sources can help you to reach that 70% fat consumption goal.

The Short Fast

Going without food can boost your ability to go into ketosis. Simply not snacking during the period between lunch and dinner can count as an intermittent fast. Any time you lower your calorie intake by not eating, you are fasting. This type of short fast can help you achieve ketosis quickly. However, fasting for longer periods of time is not advised as you could lose muscle mass.

Keto Diet Apps

Since the Keto diet has been trending, there has been a lot of attention paid to it.Both men and women are intrigued by the benefits of ketosis. Consequently, software designers are working hard to meet the demand of the Keto diet public. Apps that help track fat, protein and carb consumption are immensely popular. Also, recipe apps are fighting their way towards popularity in the app jungle. Staying in ketosis and being consistent with your meal plan, can be achieved easier by using these apps.

Tips and Tricks to Overcome Hunger and Cravings

Cravings and urges to eat foods that are not good for us, are present when we restrict the intake of foods that we are in the habit of eating. Some of our cravings are present due to emotional triggers. Here is a list of ways to overcome hunger and cravings within the framework of the Keto diet:

Chocolate

Studies have shown that a craving for chocolate may be triggered by a need for magnesium.Consequently, eating foods that are rich in magnesium can help curb your chocolate cravings.Foods that are rich in magnesium are: nuts and seeds; in particular almonds and flax seeds. You can even take a low dose of magnesium to help tame your desire.

Breads and Carbs

Lack of nitrogen can really produce a craving for bread. After a week of resisting breads that are made with white flour or wheat, you can almost feel like a crazy person; especially if you previously had a diet very high in carbs.

Learning to bake with other flours such as amaranth (which is made from a seed) or almond flour, can help you to feel more human again.

Also, eating food high in nitrogen and protein can help kill the craving for bread. .

Salty Foods

Salt consumption has long been a target for healthy diet enthusiasts. Although you need small amounts of salt to help retain some water in your body, there is no support for high levels of salt. Sometimes your salt cravings could be about silicon and chloride. Eat more nuts and seeds that contain silicon and add fish to your diet for the chloride you may be lacking in your diet.

Sugar

We experience the joy of sweet things when we are babies. Even a sugar-restricted infant can taste the sweetness of his/her mother's breast milk. We celebrate all the holidays with sugary foods, so no wonder we revere sugar as the happiest food on earth.

Don't despair, there are things you can do to curb your sugar cravings. Minerals such a carbon, phosphorous, chromium and Sulfur added to your diet, can really help with sugar withdrawal and cravings. Vegetables and cheeses can really help to add these minerals into your diet.

Watch out for artificial sweeteners as they may fill the void but they often can cause more problems than they solve.

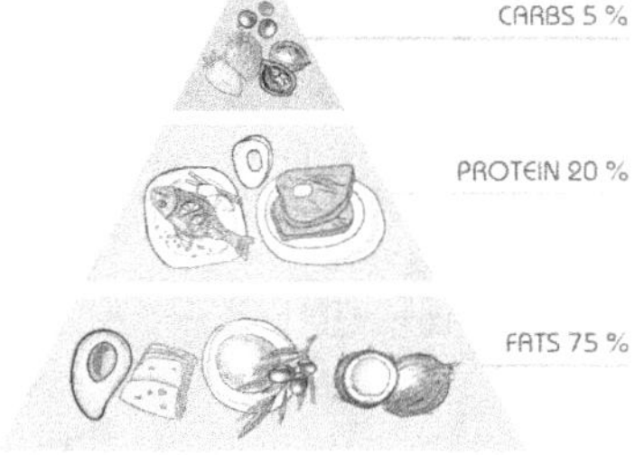

Gradually Cut Out carbs

The goal is to reduce your diet to only 5% carbs; this translates to about 25g per day. You could go cold turkey and prove to yourself that you are tough as nails; or, you can cut your carbs to a reasonable starting point of 50g and slowly work towards reducing your intake in small increments until you get to 25g.

Most times, being very aware of your food choices in the Keto diet can really be a game changer. For example, choosing to prepare a pudding made with chia seeds that has the consistency of tapioca, can easily replace a high carb processed commercial tapioca pudding; saving you many grams of carbs.

Don't Forget About fiber

Including foods with a high fiber content, can make you feel full a lot faster. We are used to thinking that foods high in grain content are our only good sources of fiber.Not true. Chia seeds, flaxseeds, coconut, pistachios, cauliflower, red cabbage, mushrooms, pecans, almonds, collard greens and pumpkin seeds are just some of the many options available on a Keto diet that will help you feel satiated.

Chapter Summary

- There are a lot of foods that can keep you on the Keto diet
- There are foods like dark chocolate that you can still have on the diet
- Taking supplements can be helpful in resisting temptations

In the next chapter you will learn about the Keto diet meal plan.

KETO MEAL PLAN AND RECIPES

THE MEAL PLAN

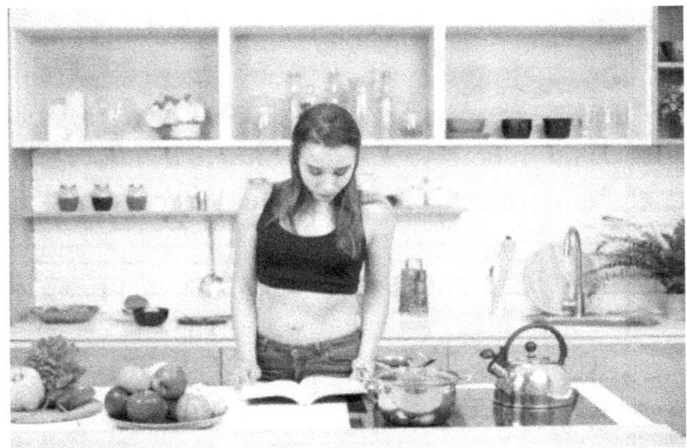

After teaching you the basics of getting into ketosis, I am so excited to present you with an example of a 14-day food plan. Since the Keto diet is not one size fits all, you will be happy to know that you can adjust the amount of food grams that are healthy for you.

For this book, I have chosen to give you recipes for each meal. I know that this can be difficult compared to other diets who just add plain meals like broiled chicken and two side vegetables to your daily meal plan. I have experienced that having exciting meals to look forward to really helped me to stick to the Keto diet. Further, I found that preparing my meals gave me a joy that I wasn't ready for.

Usually, I stayed out of the kitchen because it was such a battle-ground for me. Now, the longer I stay on the Keto diet, the more peace I have around food. I promise that the recipes I picked for your meal plan are easy to prepare. Also, do yourself a favor and shop for two weeks of the plan. Having the food available to fix through week 2, will really help you stick to the plan. And who knows, after four-teen days, you might develop a really healthy habit of cooking for yourself.

A Special Kind of Diet

I know that it seems like another type of diet would be easier to follow; but think about the value of being on a diet that is tailor-made for you. Specifically, there are extra recipes that you can replace for the recipes provided in the meal plan. Sure, it is easier to follow the cabbage diet, for instance, because all you need to worry about eating is cabbage. But how good is your body going to feel not getting all the different macronutrients that it needs? And let's be honest, a cabbage diet isn't much fun.

Further, with the resources available to us in print and on the internet, it no longer takes a person who specializes in nutrition to help you with your diet. With a little bit of brain power and good resources, you will be well on your way to health and well-being.

The Meal Plan

Day 1

- **Breakfast:** Crunchy Nutty No Grain Cereal
- **Lunch:** Cobb Salad
- **Dinner:** Meat loaf
- **Snack:** Avocado Chips

Day 2

- **Breakfast:** Berry Smoothie
- **Lunch:** Louisiana Shrimp Wraps
- **Dinner:** Garlic Pork Chops
- **Snack:** Heavenly Cheese

Day 3

- **Breakfast:** Omelet
- **Lunch:** Cauliflower Power Salad
- **Dinner:** Mahi Mahi
- **Snack:** Zucchini chips

Day 4

- **Breakfast:** Happy breakfast sandwich
- **Lunch:** Broccoli Salad
- **Dinner:** Greek Chicken
- **Snack:** Avocado Chips

Day 5

- **Breakfast:** Crunchy Nutty Whole Grain Cereal
- **Lunch:** Taco Casserole
- **Dinner:** Dinner to go
- **Snack:** Carrot cake balls

Day 6

- **Breakfast:** Eggs in pepper
- **Lunch:** Butter Shrimp
- **Dinner:** Italian Zoodles
- **Snack:** Avocado chips
- **Snack:** Guacamole

Day 7

- **Breakfast:** Scrambled Eggs
- **Lunch:** Lunch box #1
- **Dinner:** Homestyle Chicken
- **Snack:** Brussels sprouts

Week 2 Meal Plan

Day 8

- **Breakfast:** Avocado
- **Lunch:** Bacon rolls
- **Dinner:** Cali-salad
- **Snack:** Cookie dough balls

Day 9

- **Breakfast:** Happy breakfast sandwich
- **Lunch:** Cali Power
- **Dinner:** Roast chicken
- **Snack:** Bagel
- **Snack:** Guacamole

Day 10

- **Breakfast:** Pork cups
- **Lunch:** Cobb Salad
- **Dinner:** Bacon rolls
- **Snack:** Avocado balls
- **Snack:** Carrot cake balls

Day 11

- **Breakfast:** Cloud eggs

- **Lunch:** Beautiful Bacon
- **Dinner:** Meatloaf
- **Snack:** Cookie dough

Day 12

- **Breakfast:** Chocolate
- **Lunch:** Stuffed Peppers
- **Dinner:** Bacon fish
- **Snack:** Zucchini chips

Day 13

- **Breakfast:** Muffins
- **Lunch:** Stuffed Tomatoes
- **Dinner:** Salmon to go
- **Snack:** Cookie dough balls

Day 14

- **Breakfast:** Pork cups
- **Lunch:** Southwest Stuffed Avocados
- **Dinner:** Bacon rolls
- **Snack:** Avocado balls
- **Snack:** Carrot cake balls

Shopping List

- Almond
- Almond butter
- Almond flour
- Almond milk
- Asparagus (1lb.)
- Avocado, large (13pcs.)
- Baby spinach (1 bag)

- Bacon, center cut (2lbs.)
- Baking powder
- Baking soda
- Basil, fresh
- Bell pepper, green (2pcs.)
- Bell pepper, orange (2pcs.)
- Bell pepper, red (1pc.)
- Black frost Delhi ham (1lb.)
- Blue Cheese (1lb, 8oz.)
- Blueberries (1pint)
- Broccoli (3 heads)
- Brussel sprouts (1lb.)
- Butter (1 lb.)
- Carrots (1/2 lb.)
- Catfish fillets (3)
- Cauliflower (1 pc.)
- Celery
- Cheese, Monterey Jack (2lbs. shredded)
- Chia seeds
- Chicken (roasting, 5lb.)
- Chicken breasts (2lb.)
- Chicken broth
- Chicken skinless (2lb.)
- Chicken thighs (1lb.)
- Chili powder
- Chocolate chips, dark (16oz.)
- Cilantro (2 bunch)
- cinnamon
- Coconut Oil
- Colby Cheese (2lb.)
- Cooking spray (Olive oil)
- Crabmeat (12 oz. canned)
- Cream of tartar
- Cumin
- Dijon mustard

- Dried oregano
- Eggs (4dz)
- English cucumbers
- Extra-virgin olive oil
- Flax seeds
- Garlic (2 heads)
- Garlic powder
- Greek yogurt (16oz.)
- Green Onion (2 bunch)
- Ground black pepper
- Ground cloves
- Ground nutmeg
- Heavy cream (4oz.)
- Iceberg lettuce (1pc.)
- Italian seasoning
- Ketchup
- Kosher salt
- Lemon (Large, 4pcs.)
- Limes (2pcs.)
- Louisiana type hot sauce
- Mahi Fillets (4pcs.)
- Mayonnaise
- Mozzarella Cheese (2lb, 8oz.)
- Mushroom (1lb.)
- Onion dip
- Onion Powder
- Onion, diced
- Onion, dried (1 packet)
- Paprika for garnish
- Parmesan Cheese, grated (1lb.)
- Pecans (8oz.)
- Provolone Cheese (1lb, 8oz.)
- Pure vanilla extract
- Ranch seasoning (2 packets)
- Red onion (3pcs.)

- Red pepper flakes
- Red wine
- Ricotta cheese
- Romano Cheese (shredded, 10oz.)
- Salmon (8oz.)
- Shredded unsweetened coconut
- Shrimp (1lb.)
- Sour cream
- Stone ground mustard
- Strawberries
- Turkey, ground (2lbs.)
- Unsweetened cocoa powder
- Vinegar
- Walnuts (1/2 lb.)
- Zucchini (7)

Chapter Summary

Following a food plan will lead to success:

- Your meal plan needs to be tailored to your needs.
- Use tools such as a keto calendar to figure out your individual macro needs
- Cooking for each meal is worth the effort

In the next chapter you will find the recipes for your meal plan plus some extra recipes that you can switch out in your meal plan.

8

―――――

BREAKFAST RECIPES

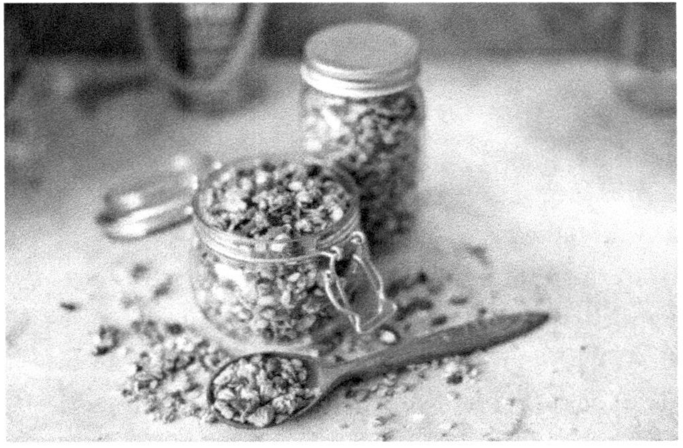

Crunchy Nutty No Grain Cereal

- Yield: 3 cups
- Prep Time: 10 minutes
- Total Time: 35 minutes

INGREDIENTS

- ¾ cup almonds, chopped
- ¾ cup walnuts, chopped
- ½ cup pecans
- ¾ cup unsweetened coconut flakes
- 2 tablespoons sesame seeds
- 2 tablespoons flax seeds
- 2 tablespoons chia seeds
- ½ teaspoon of ground cloves
- 1 ½ teaspoon ground cinnamon
- 2 teaspoons vanilla extract
- ½ teaspoon kosher salt
- 2 large egg whites
- ¼ cup melted coconut oil
- Cooking spray (olive oil)

Directions

1. Preheat oven to 350° and spray large jelly roll pan with cooking spray.
2. Using a large bowl, mix together the nuts, seeds and coconut flakes.
3. Stir in salt, cinnamon, cloves and vanilla extract.
4. In another large bowl, beat egg whites until foamy.
5. Carefully fold mixture into bowl with egg whites.
6. Add coconut oil and gently mix everything together.
7. Place nuts onto jelly roll pan – spread into one even layer.
8. Bake for 20-25 minutes or until golden brown.
9. Stir mixture at 10 minutes.
10. Cool completely.
11. Store in airtight container.

Nutrition Facts

- Servings: 8
- Amount per serving

- Calories 263
- % Daily Value*
- **Total Fat 22.6g29%**
- Saturated Fat 3.7g 18%
- Cholesterol 0mg 0%
- Sodium 53mg 2%
- Total Carbohydrate 9.4g 3%
- Dietary Fiber 6.7g24%
- Total Sugars 0.6g
- **Protein 8.9g**
- Vitamin D 0mcg0%
- Calcium 119mg9%
- Iron 2mg11%
- Potassium 221mg 5%

~

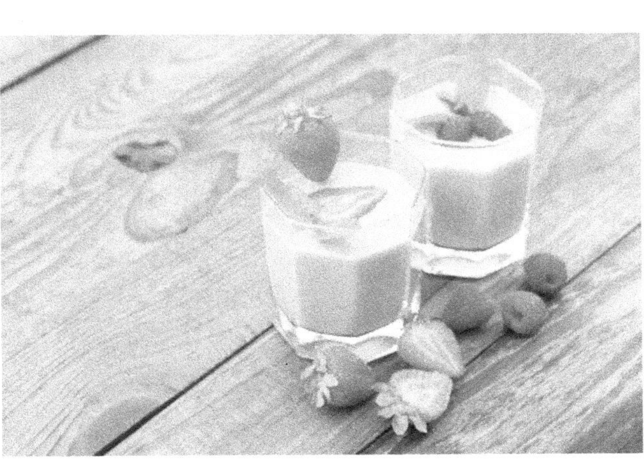

Berry Good Morning Smoothie

- Yield: 4 Servings
- Prep Time: 0 Hours 5 Minutes
- Total Time: 0 Hours 10 Minutes

Ingredients

- 1 ½ cup Strawberries, sliced in half
- 1 ½ cup raspberries, whole
- 1 cup blueberries
- 2 cups almond milk
- 1 cup baby spinach
- 4 ice cubes
- ¼ water
- Unsweetened flake coconut for garnish

Directions

1. Place ice in blender.
2. Pour in water and let sit for one minute.
3. In blender put in all ingredients except for the coconut flakes.
4. Blend together.
5. Divide between 4 cups and top with coconut flakes.

Nutrition Facts

- Servings: 4
- Amount per serving
- Calories 344
- % Daily Value*
- **Total Fat 29.7g 38%**
- Saturated Fat 25.8g 129%
- Cholesterol 0mg 0%
- Sodium 25mg 1%
- **Total Carbohydrate 22g 8%**
- Dietary Fiber 7.9g 28%
- Total Sugars 12.4g
- **Protein 4.2g**
- Vitamin D 0mcg 0%

- Calcium 47mg4%
- Iron 3mg19%
- Potassium 542mg 12%

~

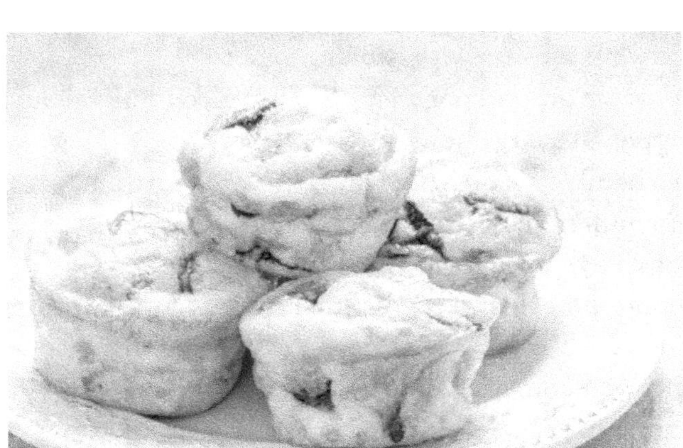

Breakfast Pork Cups

- Yield: 12 Servings
- Prep Time: 0 Hours 15 Minutes
- Total Time: 0 Hours 40 Minutes

Ingredients

- 2 lb. ground pork
- 3 cloves garlic, minced
- 1/2 tsp. paprika
- 1/2 tsp. ground cumin
- 1 tsp sea salt
- ½ tsp. black pepper
- 2 1/2 c. chopped fresh spinach
- 1 c. shredded Colby cheddar
- 12 eggs

- 1 tbsp. freshly chopped chives
- Cooking spray

Directions

1. Preheat Oven to 400⁰.
2. Spray muffin cup with cooking spray.
3. Combine ground pork, garlic, paprika, cumin, salt and pepper, in a large bowl.
4. Use hand to scoop a portion of pork mixture and press into muffin tins, creating a cup.
5. Combine spinach and cheese in a medium bowl.
6. Spoon spinach and cheese mixture into cup, leaving room for egg.
7. Crack egg into each muffin space and season with salt and pepper to taste, if desired.
8. Bake for 25 minutes until eggs are set and sausage is cooked.
9. Take out of oven and sprinkle with chives.
10. Serve immediately.

Nutrition Facts

- Servings: 12
- Amount per serving
- Calories 212
- % Daily Value*
- Total Fat 10.1g 13%
- Saturated Fat 4.2g21%
- Cholesterol 228mg 76%
- Sodium 323mg 14%
- **Total Carbohydrate 1.2g0%**
- Dietary Fiber 0.2g 1%
- Total Sugars 0.4g
- **Protein 27.8g**

- Vitamin D 15mcg77%
- Calcium 102mg8%
- Iron 2mg11%
- Potassium 433mg 9%

~

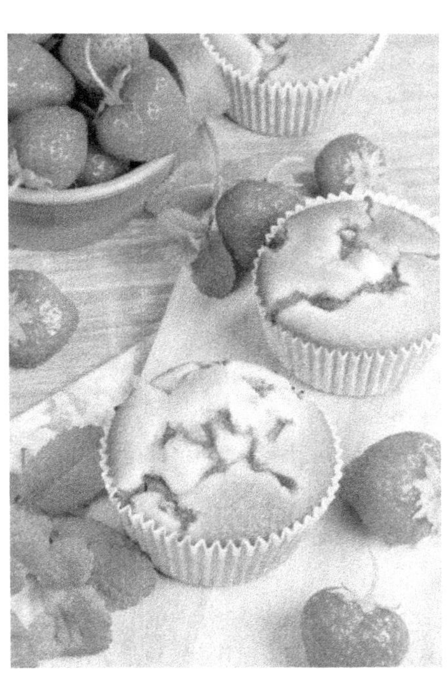

Strawberry Sunshine Muffins

- Yield: 1 Dozen
- Prep Time: 0 Hours 15 Minutes
- Total Time: 0 Hours 40 Minutes

Ingredients

- 2 1/2 c. almond flour
- 1/3 c. keto friendly sugar (such as Stevia)
- 1 1/2 tsp. baking powder

- 1/2 tsp. baking soda
- 1/2 tsp. salt
- 1/3 c. melted butter
- 1/3 c. unsweetened almond milk
- 3 large eggs
- 1 tsp. pure vanilla extract
- 2/3 c. fresh strawberries
- Zest of 1/2 lemon (optional)
- Cooking spray or cupcake liners

Directions

1. Preheat Oven to 350°.
2. Spray cooking spray on muffin tin (12) or use cupcake liners.
3. Using a large bowl, sift almond flour, sweetener, baking powder, baking soda and salt, together.
4. Gently mix in melted butter, almond milk, eggs and vanilla until combined.
5. Carefully fold in strawberries and lemon zest until well combined.
6. Using a cookie scoop, scoop batter into each muffin.
7. Bake for 20-24 minutes until golden brown – checking at 20 minutes to see if muffins are done.
8. Use toothpick test to see if done (stick a toothpick in the middle of muffin and if comes out dry, muffin is ready – if not put back in oven checking every 2 minutes).
9. Take out of oven and let cool before serving.

Nutrition Facts

- Servings: 12
- Amount per serving
- Calories 235
- % Daily Value*

- **Total Fat 17.6g 23%**
- Saturated Fat 4.5g22%
- Cholesterol 60mg 20%
- Sodium 217mg 9%
- **Total Carbohydrate 11.4g 4%**
- Dietary Fiber 2.7g 10%
- Total Sugars 5.9g
- **Protein 6.7g**
- Vitamin D 8mcg 40%
- Calcium 45mg3%
- Iron 0mg2%
- Potassium 100mg 2%

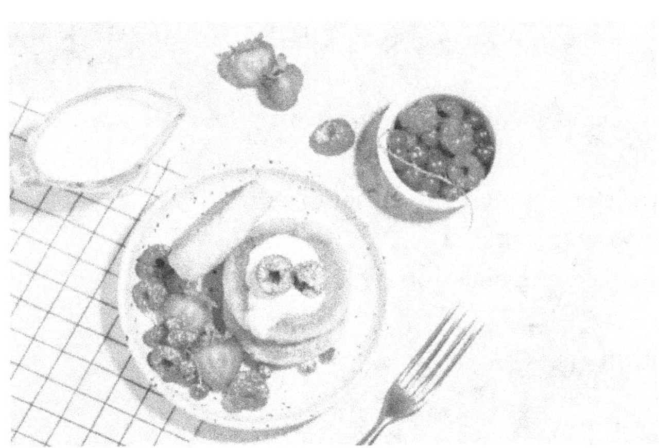

Cream Cheese Pancakes

- Yield: 8 small pancakes or 4 large pancakes
- Prep Time: 0 Hours 5 Minutes
- Total Time: 0 Hours 15 Minutes

Ingredients

- 1/2 c. almond flour
- 4 oz. cream cheese, softened
- 4 large eggs
- 1 teaspoon lemon juice
- Butter, for serving
- Cooking spray (olive oil)
- ½ cup strawberries, sliced

Directions

1. In a large bowl, mix together almond flour, cream cheese, lemon juice and eggs to make pancake batter.
2. Spray nonstick skillet with cooking spray (do this each time you add batter) and place over medium heat.
3. Using small pitcher, pour out ¼ cup of batter onto skillet.
4. Cook for 2 minutes or until edges forms and the batter bubbles.
5. Flip pancake and wait 2 more minutes until pancake is stable.
6. Transfer to plate in oven set to warm.
7. Serve with butter.
8. Garnish with sliced strawberries.

Nutrition Facts

- Servings: 2
- Amount per serving
- Calories 572
- % Daily Value*
- **Total Fat 48.9g 63%**
- Saturated Fat 20.2g 101%
- Cholesterol 450mg 150%
- Sodium 360mg 16%
- **Total Carbohydrate 11.1g 4%**
- Dietary Fiber 3.7g 13%

- Total Sugars 2.7g
- **Protein 23.2g**
- Vitamin D 39mcg195%
- Calcium 106mg8%
- Iron 3mg15%
- Potassium 261mg 6%

~

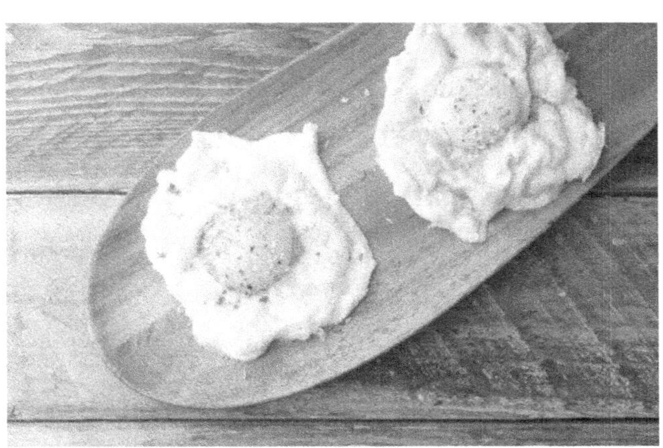

High in the Clouds Eggs

- Yields: 4 Servings
- Prep Time: 0 Hours 15 Minutes
- Total Time: 0 Hours 20 Minutes

Ingredients

- 8 large eggs
- 5 oz package grated Romano cheese
- 1/2 lb. deli turkey, chopped
- Sea Salt (too taste)
- Freshly ground black pepper (to taste)
- 2 green onions, sliced into rings for garnish

- Cooking spray (olive oil)

Directions

1. Preheat Oven to 450⁰.
2. Spray large cookie sheet with cooking spray.
3. Separate egg yolk and egg white (placing egg whites in a medium bowl and egg yolks in medium bowl).
4. Using a hand mixer, beat egg whites into stiff peaks (about 3 minutes).
5. Fold in Romano cheese, turkey and salt and pepper to taste.
6. Gently spoon 8 mounds of egg whites onto cookie sheet.
7. Indent center of egg white mounds to make room for egg yolk.
8. Gently spoon yolk into the middle of egg white (do this for the rest).
9. Bake until yolks are set (3-4 minutes).
10. Place green onions slices on top of each mound
11. Serve immediately.

Nutrition Facts

- Servings: 8
- Amount per serving
- Calories 156
- % Daily Value*
- **Total Fat 9.4g 12%**
- Saturated Fat 3.9g19%
- Cholesterol 215mg 72%
- Sodium 602mg 26%
- **Total Carbohydrate 3.4g1%**
- Dietary Fiber 0.2g 1%
- Total Sugars 1.7g
- **Protein 14.4g**

- Vitamin D 18mcg88%
- Calcium 175mg13%
- Iron 2mg10%
- Potassium 188mg 4%

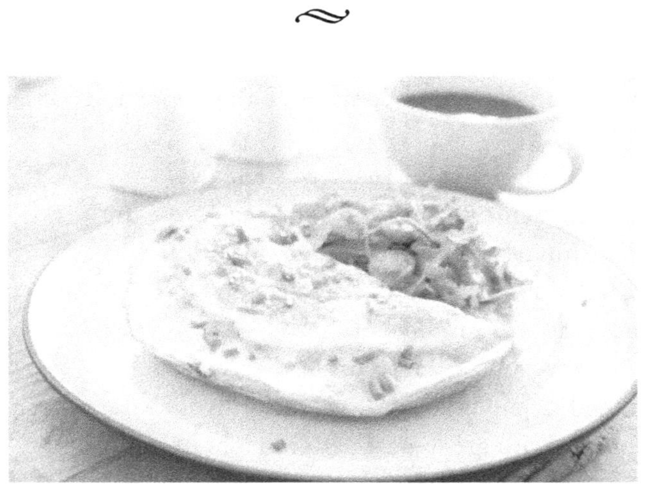

Shake 'em up Omelets

- Yields: 2
- Prep Time: 0 Hours 10 Minutes
- Total Time: 0 Hours 15 Minutes

Ingredients

- nonstick cooking spray (olive oil)
- 4 large eggs
- 2/3 c. shredded Colby Cheese
- 1/2 Red onion, finely chopped
- 1/2 c. Black Forest deli ham, diced
- 1 green bell pepper, chopped
- ½ cup Spinach
- Sea salt (to taste)

- Freshly ground black pepper (to taste)
- ¼ cup green onion, chopped

Directions

1. Spray 2 16oz mason jars liberally with cooking spray.
2. Break two eggs into each mason jar.
3. Divide cheese, onion, ham and bell pepper and spinach in half.
4. Place divided mix into each mason jar.
5. Put lids on mason jars and shake each one until everything is combined (about 1 minute).
6. REMOVE LIDS and place mason jars into the microwave and heat for 2 minutes.
7. Check every 30 seconds to see if eggs are set.
8. Using hot pad or oven mitts, carefully take out mason jars.
9. Garnish with green part of onion (chopped).
10. Serve immediately.

Nutrition Facts

- Servings: 2
- Amount per serving
- Calories 378
- % Daily Value*
- **Total Fat 25.2g 32%**
- Saturated Fat 11.7g 59%
- Cholesterol 427mg 142%
- Sodium 816mg 35%
- **Total Carbohydrate 10.4g 4%**
- Dietary Fiber 2g 7%
- Total Sugars 5.2g
- **Protein 28.2g**
- Vitamin D 35mcg175%
- Calcium 338mg26%

- Iron 3mg17%
- Potassium 473mg 10%

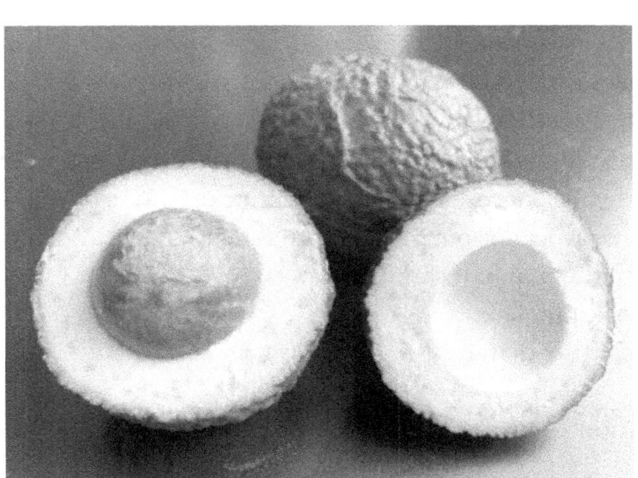

Bacon Avocado Keto Breakfast

- Yields: 4
- Prep Time: 0 Hours 10 Minutes
- Total Time: 0 Hours 20 Minutes

Ingredients

- 2 large avocados
- 1/3 c. shredded mozzarella
- 8 slices center cut bacon
- Juice of one-half lemon

Directions

1. Heat oven broil.
2. Line small jelly roll sheet with foil.

3. Cut open avocado and take out pit.
4. Carefully remove skin of avocado.
5. Sprinkle lemon juice liberally over avocado.
6. Fill each avocado half with cheese.
7. Put Avocado halves together and wrap bacon around whole avocado (4 slices each).
8. Place avocados on jelly roll sheet with foil.
9. Broil avocados until bacon is cooked (5 minutes).
10. Carefully turn avocados with tongs and cook the other side until bacon is cooked (5 minutes).
11. Take avocados out of oven (broiler).
12. Cut them in half carefully.
13. Serve on plate.
14. Eat immediately.

Nutrition Facts

- Servings: 2
- Amount per serving
- Calories 543
- % Daily Value*
- **Total Fat 47g60%**
- Saturated Fat 11.7g 59%
- Cholesterol 33mg 11%
- Sodium 460mg 20%
- **Total Carbohydrate 17.5g 6%**
- Dietary Fiber 13.5g 48%
- Total Sugars 1g
- **Protein 17.2g**
- Vitamin D 0mcg 0%
- Calcium 27mg2%
- Iron 1mg7%
- Potassium 975mg 21%

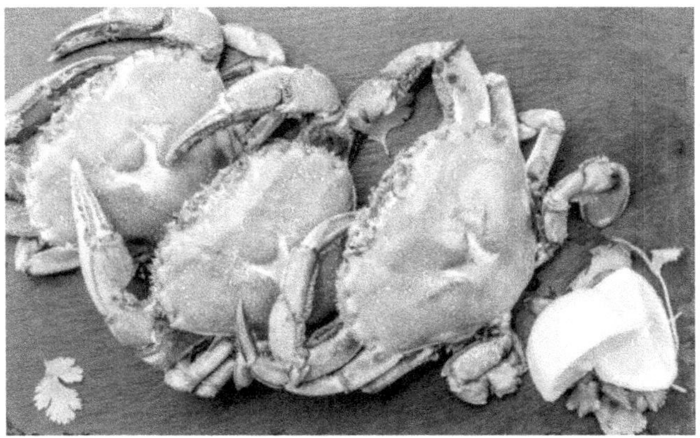

Breakfast Seafood Plate

- Yields:4
- Prep Time: 0 Hours 10 Minutes
- Total Time: 0 Hours 20 Minutes

Ingredients

- 4 large eggs
- 12 oz. canned crab meat
- 2 large avocados
- ½ cup ricotta cheese
- ½ cup red onion chopped fine
- ½ cup mayonnaise
- ½ cup spinach
- 2 tbsp. olive oil
- ½ lemon
- Red pepper flakes (to taste)
- Salt and pepper (to taste)

Directions

1. Bring a small pot filled with water to boil.

2. Carefully lower eggs (still in shell) into water
3. Boil (4-8 minutes).
4. Drain water out of the saucepan and carefully put eggs to cool.
5. Peel eggs and cut in half.
6. Slice Avocados.
7. Mix mayonnaise and onion with crab meat.
8. Arrange all ingredients on a serving platter.
9. Sprinkle olive oil over spinach and eggs.
10. Squeeze lemon half over avocado.
11. Season to taste with salt, pepper and red pepper flakes.

Nutrition Facts

- Servings: 4
- Amount per serving
- Calories 571
- % Daily Value*
- **Total Fat 45.4g 58%**
- Saturated Fat 9.6g48%
- Cholesterol 249mg 83%
- Sodium 858mg 37%
- **Total Carbohydrate 19.3g 7%**
- Dietary Fiber 6.8g 24%
- Total Sugars 2.9g
- **Protein 22.7g**
- Vitamin D 18mcg88%
- Calcium 434mg33%
- Iron 3mg16%
- Potassium 617mg 13%

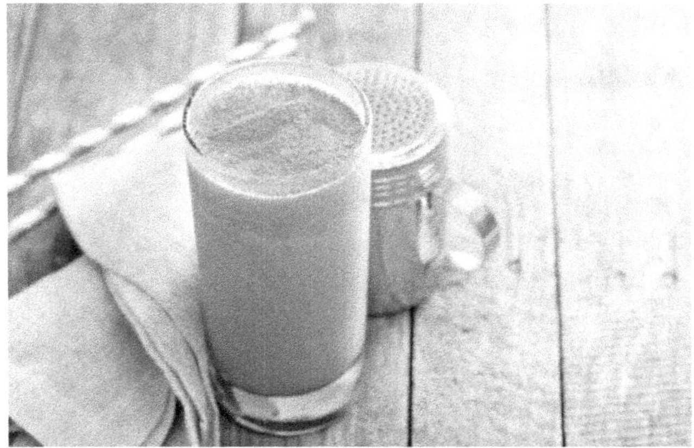

Chocolate Miracle Shake

- Yields:1
- Prep Time: 0 Hours 5 Minutes
- Total Time: 0 Hours 5 Minutes

Ingredients

- 3/4 c. almond milk
- 1/2 c. ice
- 2 tbsp. almond butter
- 2 tbsp. unsweetened cocoa powder
- 2 to 3 tbsp. keto-friendly sugar substitute (Splenda)
- 1 tbsp. chia seeds, plus more for serving
- 2 tsp. pure vanilla extract
- Pinch kosher salt

Directions

1. Add ice cubes to the blender.
2. Pour in almond milk, wait one minute for ice to begin melting (will make blending easier).
3. Add remaining ingredients.

4. Blend all ingredients for 1 minute.
5. Pour into glass.

Nutrition Facts

- Servings: 1
- Amount per serving
- Calories 934
- % Daily Value*
- **Total Fat 79.8g 102%**
- Saturated Fat 42.2g 211%
- Cholesterol 0mg 0%
- Sodium 41mg 2%
- Total Carbohydrate 46.7g 17%
- Dietary Fiber 30.2g 108%
- Total Sugars 8.7g
- **Protein 22.4g**
- Vitamin D 0mcg 0%
- Calcium 411mg32%
- Iron 15mg82%
- Potassium 1121mg 24%

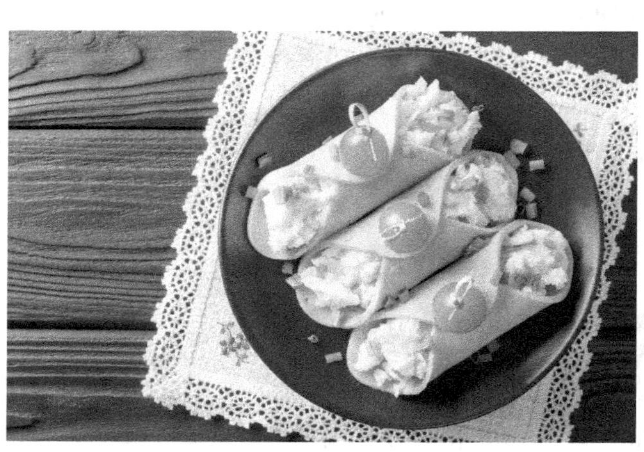

Ham and Egg Plate

- Yields: 2
- Prep Time: 0 Hours 5 Minutes
- Total Time: 0 Hours 10 Minutes

Ingredients

- 5 oz. deli ham slices, cut thick
- 4 eggs
- 2 large avocados, pitted and peeled, cut into slices
- 4 tbsp. pecans, shelled and halved
- ½ red bell pepper slices
- ½ yellow bell pepper slices
- ¼ cup red onions, sliced thinly
- Salt and pepper to taste
- 2 romaine lettuce leaves
- 2 tbsp. olive oil
- Cooking spray (olive oil)

Directions

1. Warm deli ham slices in nonstick pan.
2. Spray pan with cooking spray.
3. Place pan on medium heat.
4. Beat eggs together.
5. Pour eggs into skillet.
6. Add salt and pepper to taste.
7. Scramble eggs until set.
8. Place ham, eggs, avocado, pecans, bell peppers on large romaine leaf.
9. Serve immediately.

Nutrition Facts

- Servings: 2
- Amount per serving
- Calories 682
- % Daily Value*
- **Total Fat 54.2g 70%**
- Saturated Fat 13.1g 65%
- Cholesterol 368mg 123%
- Sodium 1062mg46%
- **Total Carbohydrate 27.9g 10%**
- Dietary Fiber 15.8g 56%
- Total Sugars 5.9g
- **Protein 27.6g**
- Vitamin D 31mcg154%
- Calcium 99mg8%
- Iron 4mg22%
- Potassium 1450mg 31%

~

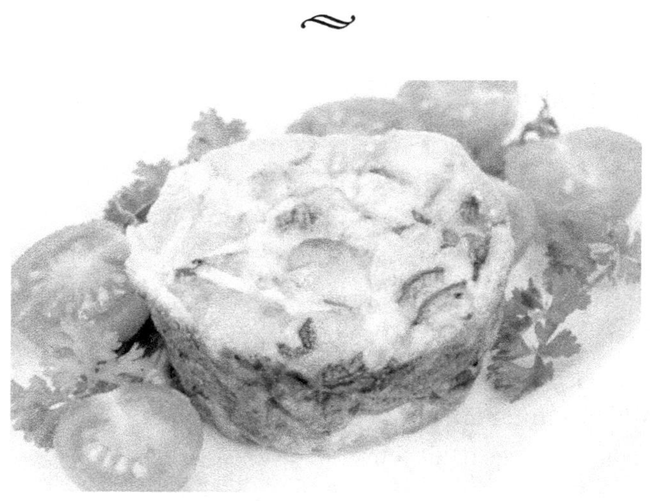

Poppin' Egg Cups

- Yields: 4-6
- Prep Time: 0 Hours 15 Minutes

- Total Time: 0 Hours 35 Minutes

Ingredients

- 12 center cut bacon
- 10 large eggs
- 1/4 c. sour cream
- 1/2 c. shredded Colby Jack Cheese
- 1/2 c. shredded mozzarella
- ½ cup white onion, chopped
- ½ cup bell pepper, chopped
- 2 jalapeños, pickled and sliced into rounds
- 1 tsp. garlic powder
- Sea salt to taste
- black pepper to taste
- 2 tbsp. butter
- nonstick cooking spray

Directions

1. Preheat oven to 375.
2. In a large nonstick skillet cook bacon over medium heat (do not let bacon crisp).
3. Drain bacon on a paper towel lined plate to absorb the fat.
4. After bacon is done, pour off most of the fat, leaving about an inch in skillet.
5. Sauté onion and bell pepper until translucent.
6. In a large bowl, whisk together eggs, bell peppers, onion, sour cream, cheeses, garlic powder and salt and pepper to taste.
7. Spray well muffin tin with cooking spray.
8. Cut bacon pieces in half.
9. Put two halves of bacon in each muffin space.
10. Pour egg mixture in each cup, leaving one inch of cup free (3/4 filled).

11. Place jalapeño slices on each muffin.
12. Bake for 20 minutes or until eggs are set.
13. Cool for 3 minutes.
14. Serve immediately.

Nutrition Facts

- Servings: 12
- Amount per serving
- Calories 127
- % Daily Value*
- **Total Fat 8.7g 11%**
- Saturated Fat 3.8g19%
- Cholesterol 169mg 56%
- Sodium 298mg 13%
- **Total Carbohydrate 1.8g1%**
- Dietary Fiber 0.3g 1%
- Total Sugars 0.9g
- **Protein 9.9g**
- Vitamin D 15mcg73%
- Calcium 65mg5%
- Iron 1mg5%
- Potassium 90mg 2%

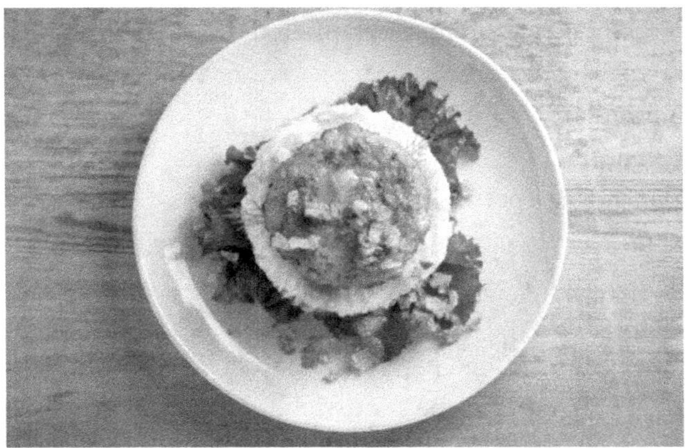

Happy Breakfast Sandwich

- Yields: 3
- Prep Time: 0 Hours 5 Minutes
- Total Time: 0 Hours 15 Minutes

Ingredients

- 6 large eggs
- 2 tbsp. heavy cream
- Pinch red pepper flakes
- Kosher salt
- Freshly ground black pepper
- 1 tbsp. butter
- 3 slices Monterey Jack Cheese
- 6 sausage patties
- Tomato, sliced

Directions

1. In a medium bowl, whisk eggs, heavy cream and red pepper flakes together.
2. Season with salt and pepper to taste.

3. Pour some egg mixture into skilled (over medium heat).
4. When the eggs are set, place a slice of cheese onto egg and let it melt for 1 minute.
5. Take out of skillet and place on plate.
6. Heat sausage patties in the skillet (2).
7. When warm place on sausage patty on the plate.
8. Put egg mixture onto the patty.
9. Place a slice of tomato on top.
10. Place other sausage patty on top to make sandwich.
11. Repeat for other three sandwiches.

Nutrition Facts

- Servings: 6
- Amount per serving
- Calories 134
- % Daily Value*
- **Total Fat 9.9g 13%**
- Saturated Fat 4.4g22%
- Cholesterol 199mg 66%
- Sodium 145mg 6%
- **Total Carbohydrate 0.7g0%**
- Dietary Fiber 0g 0%
- Total Sugars 0.7g
- **Protein 10g**
- Vitamin D 0mcg 0%
- Calcium 106mg8%
- Iron 17mg95%
- Potassium 77mg 2%

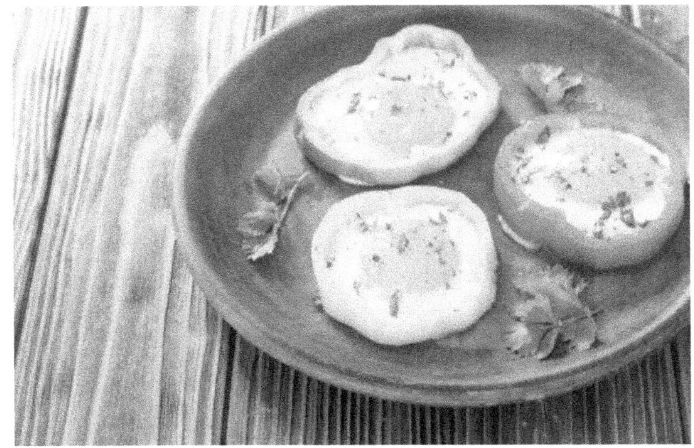

Eggs in Peppers

- Yields: 3
- Prep Time: 0 Hours 5 Minutes
- Total Time: 0 Hours 20 Minutes

Ingredients

- 1 bell pepper, sliced into ¼" rings (red, green, orange or yellow)
- 6 eggs
- Kosher salt
- Freshly ground black pepper
- 2 green peppers, chopped
- 2 tbsp. cilantro, chopped
- Cooking spray

Directions

1. Spray skillet with cooking spray.
2. Place skillet on medium heat.
3. Place bell pepper in skillet.
4. Crack egg in the middle of bell pepper ring.

5. Cook until set.
6. Flip egg and cook until done the way you like it.

Nutrition Facts

- Servings: 3
- Amount per serving
- Calories **139**
- % Daily Value*
- **Total Fat 8.9g 11%**
- Saturated Fat 2.7g **14%**
- **Cholesterol** 327mg **109%**
- **Sodium** 175mg **8%**
- **Total Carbohydrate** 3.7g **1%**
- Dietary Fiber 0.5g **2%**
- Total Sugars 2.7g
- **Protein** 11.5g
- Vitamin D 31mcg 154%
- Calcium 50mg 4%
- Iron 2mg 10%
- Potassium 193mg 4%

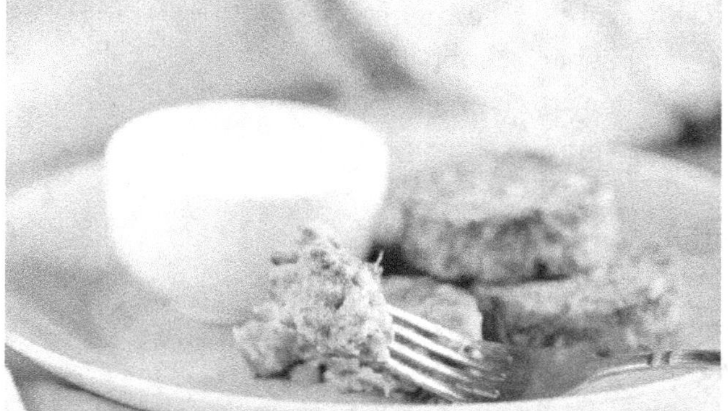

Zucchini Cups

- Yields: 12
- Prep Time: 0 Hours 10Minute
- Total Time: 0 Hours 40 Minutes

Ingredients

- Cooking spray, for pan
- 2 zucchini, cut in circles
- 1/4 lb. ham, chopped
- 1/2 c. tomato, diced
- 8 eggs
- 1/2 c. heavy cream
- Kosher salt
- Freshly ground black pepper
- ¼ c. fresh basil, chopped
- 1Pinch red pepper flakes
- 1 c. shredded cheddar

Directions

1. Preheat Oven to 400°.
2. Spray muffin tin with cooking spray.
3. Place zucchini round on bottom of muffin cup.
4. Add ham and tomato to each muffin cup.
5. In a medium bowl, beat eggs together.
6. Add heavy cream, basil and red paper.
7. Season with salt and pepper to taste.
8. Pour egg mixture over ham and tomato.
9. Top each muffin cup with cheese.
10. Bake until eggs are set (30 minutes).

Nutrition Facts

- Servings: 12
- **Amount per serving**
- **Calories 98**
- **% Daily Value***
- **Total Fat** 6.3g **8%**
- Saturated Fat 2.8g **14%**
- **Cholesterol** 123mg 41%
- **Sodium** 239mg 10%
- **Total Carbohydrate** 2.3g **1%**
- Dietary Fiber 0.6g **2%**
- Total Sugars 1.1g
- **Protein 8.1g**
- Vitamin D 13mcg 64%
- Calcium 67mg 5%
- Iron 1mg 5%
- Potassium 182mg 4%

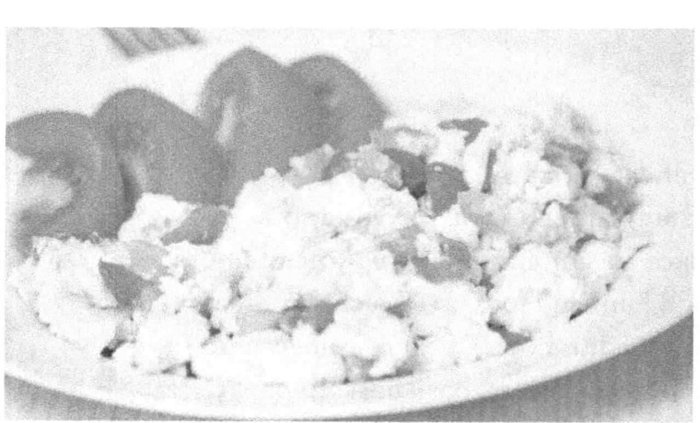

Quick Scrambled Eggs

Ingredients

- 4 eggs

- 2 tbls. Butter
- ¼ c. onion
- ½ c. cherry tomatoes, halved
- ¼ c. pickled jalapeno slices (optional)

Directions

1. In a medium skillet, heat butter over medium heat.
2. In a small bowl beat eggs.
3. Add onion and sauté until translucent.
4. Add beaten egg, tomatoes and jalapeño.
5. Stir egg mixture until it is set.
6. Serve immediately.

Nutrition Facts

- **Servings: 2**
- **Amount per serving**
- **Calories 176**
- **% Daily Value***
- **Total Fat** 12.9g **17%**
- Saturated Fat 5.3g **27%**
- **Cholesterol** 338mg **113%**
- **Sodium** 155mg **7%**
- **Total Carbohydrate** 3.8g **1%**
- Dietary Fiber 0.9g **3%**
- Total Sugars 2.5g
- **Protein** 11.7g
- Vitamin D 34mcg 168%
- Calcium 56mg 4%
- Iron 2mg 10%
- Potassium 247mg 5%

9

———

LUNCH RECIPES

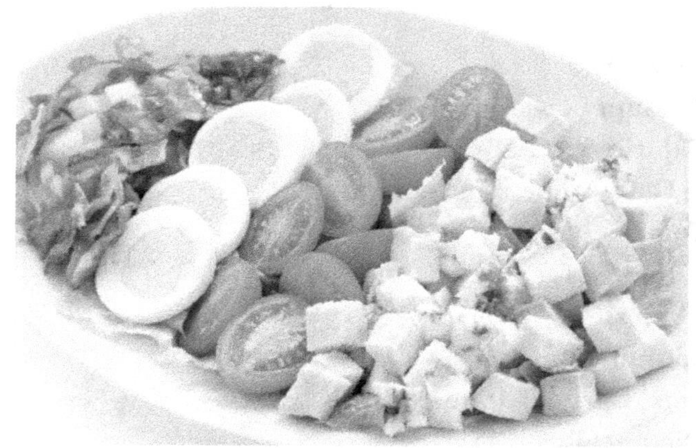

Cobb Salad

- Yields: 8 Servings
- Prep Time: 0 Hours 15 Minutes
- Total Time: 0 Hours 20 Minutes

Ingredients

- 3 tbsp. mayonnaise
- 3 tbsp. Greek yogurt
- 2 tbsp. white wine vinegar
- 1 tsp. Dijon mustard
- Sea salt (to taste)
- black pepper (to taste)
- 6 hard-boiled eggs, quartered
- 6 strips bacon, cooked crisp,
- 6 oz. breast of chicken, grilled (or baked)
- 1 large avocado, diced
- 1/2 c. crumbled blue cheese
- 1 c. cherry tomatoes, halved,
- 2 tbsp. green onions, chopped
- 1 small head iceberg lettuce roughly chopped

Directions

1. In a medium bowl, whisk together mayonnaise, yogurt, vinegar, mustard, salt and pepper to taste.
2. Using a large shallow bowl arrange salad as follows:lettuce on the bottom, place other ingredients in rows on top of lettuce.
3. Drizzle dressing over arranged salad.

Nutrition Facts

- Servings: 8
- Amount per serving
- Calories 321
- % Daily Value*
- **Total Fat 20.6g 26%**
- Saturated Fat 7.2g36%
- Cholesterol 166mg 55%
- Sodium 580mg 25%
- **Total Carbohydrate 8.2g3%**

- Dietary Fiber 2g 7%
- Total Sugars 4.4g
- **Protein 25.8g**
- Vitamin D 12mcg58%
- Calcium 150mg12%
- Iron 1mg7%
- Potassium 475mg 10%

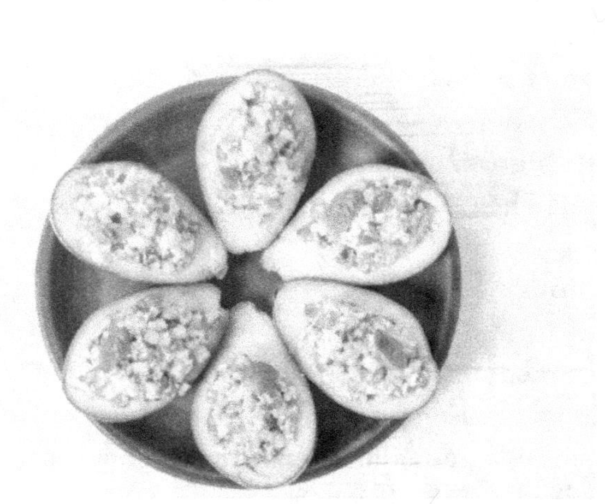

Southwest Stuffed Avocados

- Yields: 4-8 Servings
- PrepTime: 0 Hours 10 Minutes
- Total Time: 0 Hours 25 Minutes

Ingredients

- 4 large avocados
- Juice of 1 lime
- 1 tbsp. extra-virgin olive oil
- 1 medium onion, chopped
- 1 lb. ground turkey

- 2 tbsp. Homemade Taco seasoning*(see below)
- Kosher salt and black pepper to taste
- 2/3 c. shredded Colby Jack cheese
- 1/2 c. shredded iceberg lettuce
- 1/2 c. roma tomatoes, chopped
- ½ cup Sour cream
- 3 tablespoons Greek Yogurt

Directions

1. Pit and peel avocados and cut in half.
2. Scoop a little of avocado to make a deeper well for other ingredients.
3. Put aside the avocado that you scooped out.
4. Squeeze lime juice over avocado to preserve avocado.
5. Brown turkey meat in a nonstick skillet over medium heat.
6. Add taco seasoning and onion to meat mixture.
7. Combine well with ground turkey, making sure to crumble meat.
8. Finish cooking ground turkey until no longer pink (5 minutes).
9. Cook meat for 2 minutes.
10. Scoop meat into the hollowed-out middle of avocado.
11. Mix sour cream and Greek yogurt.
12. Top avocado with sour cream mixture.
13. Top each avocado half with a portion of lettuce, cheese and tomato.
14. Add a tablespoon of sour cream mixture to each stuffed avocado.
15. Serve immediately.

***Homemade Taco Seasoning**

Ingredients

- 6 tablespoons chili powder
- 2 1/2 tablespoons cumin
- 1 ½ tablespoon paprika
- 1 tablespoon salt
- 1 ½ teaspoon garlic powder
- 1 teaspoon dried onion
- 1 teaspoon oregano
- 1 teaspoon black pepper

Directions

1. Mix ingredients together in jar or mall bowl.
2. Store in airtight container.

Nutrition Facts

- Servings: 4
- Amount per serving
- Calories 889
- % Daily Value*
- **Total Fat 73.2g 94%**
- Saturated Fat 22.2g 111%
- Cholesterol 166mg 55%
- Sodium 374mg 16%
- **Total Carbohydrate 23.5g 9%**
- Dietary Fiber 14.4g 51%
- Total Sugars 3.5g
- **Protein 45.9g**
- Vitamin D 4mcg 21%
- Calcium 358mg28%
- Iron 4mg22%
- Potassium 1479mg 31%

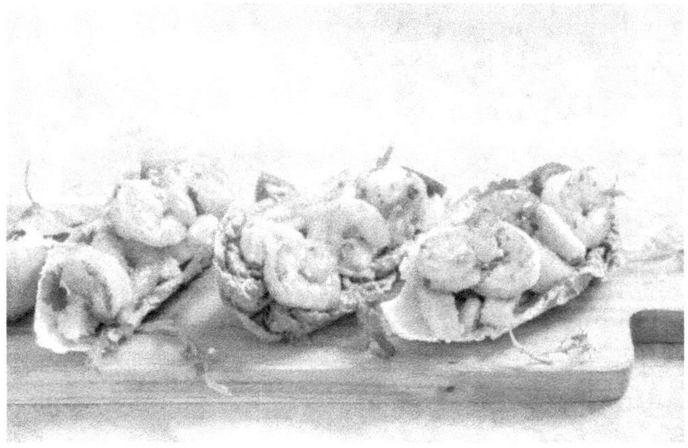

Louisiana Shrimp Wraps

- Yields: 4
- Prep Time: 0 Hours 15 Minutes
- Cook Time: 0 Hours 20 Minutes
- Total Time: 0 Hours 35 Minutes

Ingredients
Sauce:

- 2 tbsp. butter
- 3 garlic cloves, minced
- 1/2 c. Louisiana type hot sauce

Shrimp:

- 1 tbsp. extra-virgin olive oil
- 1 lb. shrimp, peeled and deveined, tails removed
- Sea salt and pepper, to taste

Wrap:

- 1 head butter lettuce, leaves separated

- 1/2 red onion, finely chopped
- ½ cup celery, chopped fine
- 1/2 c. blue cheese, crumbled

Directions
Sauce:

1. Melt butter in a small saucepan, over medium heat.
2. Add garlic and sauté for (2 minutes).
3. Add hot sauce and combine with butter and garlic.
4. Turn down heat to low.

Shrimp:

1. Add oil to a large skillet on medium heat for (1 minute).
2. Add shrimp and season with salt and pepper, cook (3 minutes).
3. With spoon or spatula, flip shrimp to the other side (3 minutes).
4. Cook until shrimp is pink and opaque.
5. Remove from heat.

Wraps:

1. Take one whole leaf of butter lettuce and fill with shrimp.
2. Top with equally divided portions of red onion, celery and blue cheese.
3. Serve immediately.

Nutrition Information

- Servings: 4
- Amount per serving
- Calories 288
- % Daily Value*

- **Total Fat 16.1g 21%**
- Saturated Fat 7.9g40%
- Cholesterol 267mg 89%
- Sodium 565mg 25%
- **Total Carbohydrate 4.9g2%**
- Dietary Fiber 0.6g 2%
- Total Sugars 1g
- **Protein 29.9g**
- Vitamin D 4mcg 20%
- Calcium 206mg16%
- Iron 1mg5%

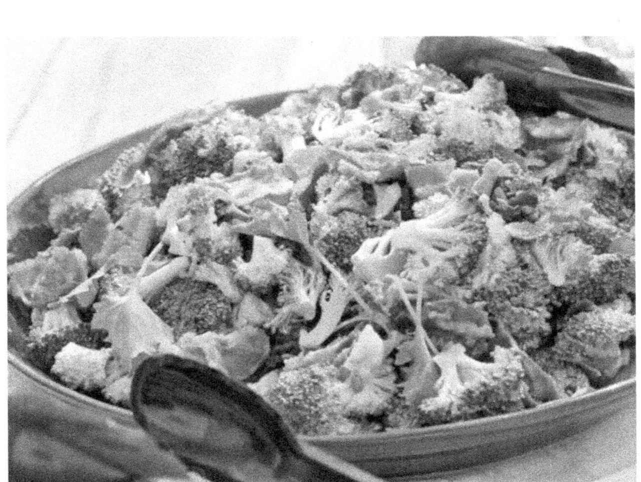

Super Broccoli Salad

- Yields: 4 Servings
- Prep Time: 0 Hours 15 Minutes
- Total Time: 0 Hours 35 Minutes

Ingredients

- 2 heads broccoli, cut into bite-size florets
- 1/2 c. shredded Colby Jack
- 1/2 red onion, thinly sliced
- 1/4 c. toasted sliced almonds
- 4 slices bacon, cooked and crumbled
- ½ cup green onion, chopped
- 2 tsp sea salt (for water)

Dressing

- 2/3 c. mayonnaise
- 3 tbsp. red wine vinegar
- 1 1/2 tbsp. stone ground mustard
- Salt and pepper to taste

Directions

1. Blanch Broccoli.
2. Put 5 cups of water in a large saucepan and bring to a boil.
3. Place broccoli florets in boiling salted water and let them cook until they are tender (3 minutes).
4. Prepare a large bowl with water and ice.
5. Drain broccoli from saucepan by using a colander.
6. Plunge drained broccoli into ice water "bath" Leave in for 5 minutes.
7. Meanwhile prepare the dressing.
8. In a mason jar with lid, add vinegar, stone ground mustard, salt and pepper to taste.Put on lid and shake vigorously until dressing is combined well.

Salad

1. Place broccoli, onion, almonds, and bacon in a large serving bowl.
2. Toss to mix ingredients.

3. Pour dressing over salad and coat well.
4. Refrigerate until serving time.

Nutrition Information

- Calories 378
- % Daily Value*
- **Total Fat 29g37%**
- Saturated Fat 7.7g39%
- Cholesterol 46mg 15%
- Sodium 849mg 37%
- **Total Carbohydrate 16.8g 6%**
- Dietary Fiber 2.5g 9%
- Total Sugars 4.5g
- **Protein 13.8g**
- Vitamin D 2mcg 9%
- Calcium 160mg12%
- Iron 1mg7%
- Potassium 375mg 8%

~

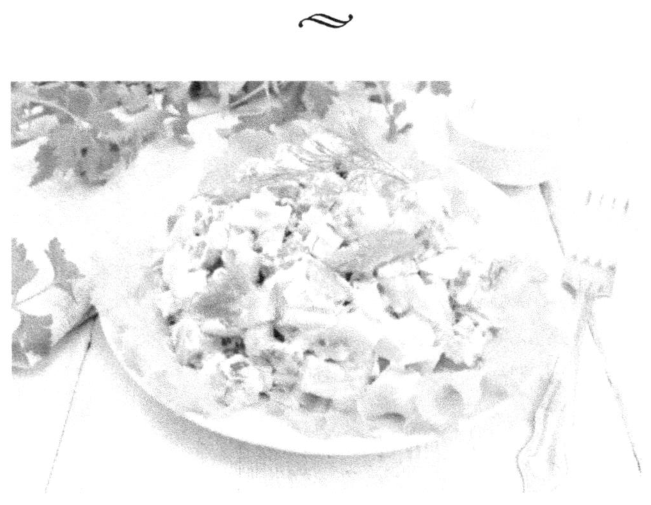

Egg Salad Delight

- Prep Time: 0 Hours 15 Minutes
- Total Time: 0 Hours 25 Minutes

Ingredients

- 2 tbsp. mayonnaise
- 1 tbsp. Greek yogurt
- 2 tsp. lemon juice
- ¼ cup red onion, chopped fine
- ¼ cup celery, chopped fine
- ½ teaspoon celery salt
- Salt pepper to taste
- 6 hard-boiled eggs, peeled and chopped
- 1 large avocado, cubed
- ¼ cup shredded iceberg lettuce, for topping
- 4 slices crisp cooked bacon for topping

Directions

1. In deep bowl, mix together mayonnaise, yogurt, lemon juice, onions, celery salt and celery.
2. Season with salt and pepper to taste.
3. Add egg and avocado and gently combine with dressing.
4. Serve individually and top with shredded lettuce and bacon.
5. Store remaining egg salad in sealed container.

Nutrition Information

- Calories 343
- % Daily Value*
- **Total Fat 27g35%**
- Saturated Fat 7.2g 36%
- Cholesterol 270mg90%
- Sodium 600mg26%

- **Total Carbohydrate 8.5g 3%**
- Dietary Fiber 3.7g13%
- Total Sugars 2.1g
- **Protein 18g**
- Vitamin D 23mcg116%
- Calcium 64mg5%
- Iron 2mg11%
- Potassium 489mg 10%

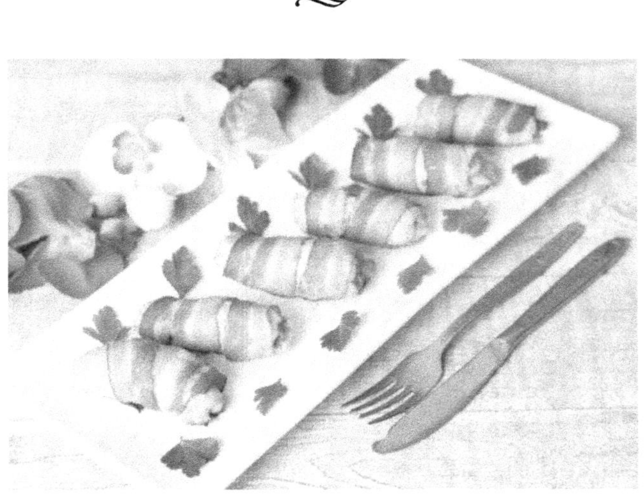

Marvelous Bacon Rolls

- Yields: 12
- Prep Time: 0 Hours 10 Minutes
- Total Time: 0 Hours 30 Minutes

Ingredients

- 6 slices center cut bacon, halved
- 2 English cucumbers, thinly sliced
- 2 medium carrots, thinly sliced

- 1 large avocado, diced
- 4 oz. cream cheese, softened
- 1 teaspoon paprika for garnish

Directions

1. In a nonstick skillet over medium heat, cook bacon slices until they are pliable and not crunchy.
2. In large bowl, mix, cucumbers, carrots and avocado.
3. Take a halved bacon slices and lay out on cutting board.Spread the length of bacon with cream cheese.
4. Add 1 tablespoon of cucumber mixture to bacon and starting at one end, carefully roll up bacon tightly.May use toothpick to secure.
5. Garnish tops of bacon roll with paprika.

Diet Information

- Calories 130
- % Daily Value*
- **Total Fat 10.6g 14%**
- Saturated Fat 4.1g20%
- Cholesterol 21mg 7%
- Sodium 256mg 11%
- **Total Carbohydrate 4.7g2%**
- Dietary Fiber 1.6g 6%
- Total Sugars 1.4g
- **Protein 5g**
- Vitamin D 0mcg 0%
- Calcium 22mg2%
- Iron 1mg3%
- Potassium 252mg 5%

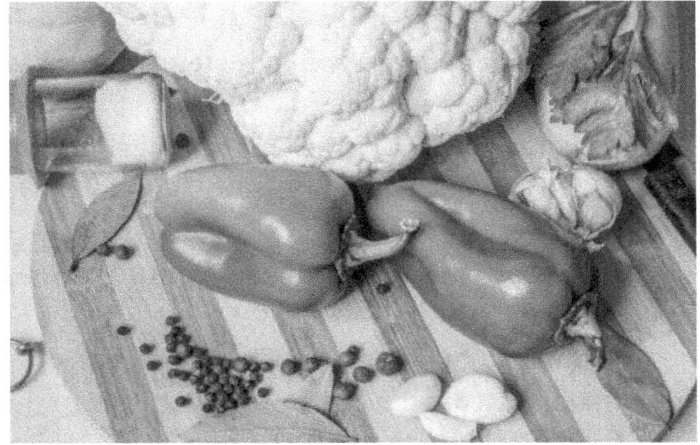

Cauliflower Power Salad

- Yields: 6 Servings
- Prep Time: 0 Hours 10 Minutes
- Total Time: 0 Hours 30 Minutes

Ingredients

- 1 large cauliflower, cut into florets
- 6 slices of bacon
- 1/2 cup mayonnaise
- ½ cup plain Greek yogurt
- ½ cup p 1 tbsp. lemon juice
- 1/2 tsp. garlic powder
- 1 tbsp. Salt (for boiling water)
- Sea salt and pepper to taste
- 1 1/2 c. shredded Monterey jack cheese
- ½ cup tomato, seeded and diced
- ½ cup red bell pepper, diced
- ¼ cup red onion, diced
- ¼ cup green onions, sliced

Directions

1. In large saucepan, bring six cups of water and salt to boil.
2. Add cauliflower florets into boiling water cover and coop for 4 minutes or until tender.
3. Using a colander, drain florets from the water and place on a cookie sheet lined with paper towels.Dry cauliflower.
4. Roughly chop cauliflower.
5. Using a large bowl mix together geek yogurt, mayonnaise, lemon juice and garlic powder.
6. Add cauliflower, tomato, bell pepper, onions, and olives and coat well with dressing.
7. Top with bacon, cheese and green onions.
8. Refrigerate until serving.

Nutrition Facts

- Servings: 4
- Amount per serving
- Calories 406
- % Daily Value*
- **Total Fat 20.6g 26%**
- Saturated Fat 6g 30%
- Cholesterol 48mg 16%
- Sodium 766mg 33%
- **Total Carbohydrate 23.2g 8%**
- Dietary Fiber 2.7g 10%
- Total Sugars 12.4g
- Protein 32.3g
- Vitamin D omcg 0%
- Calcium 282mg22%
- Iron 1mg5%
- Potassium 646mg 14%

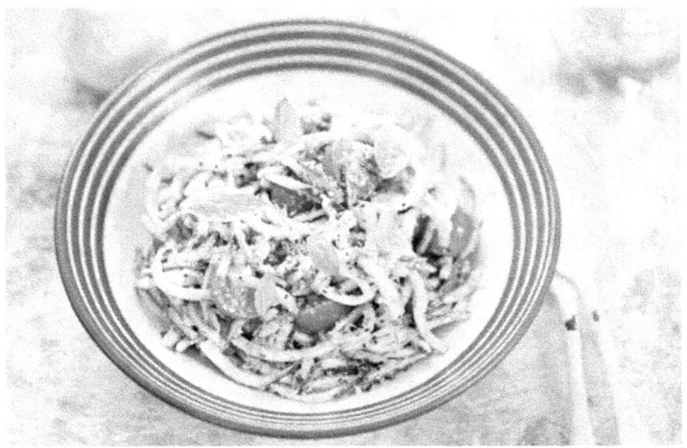

Italian Zoodles

- Yields: 4
- Prep Time: 0 Hours 10 Minutes
- Total Time: 0 Hours 25 Minutes

Ingredients

- 4 large zucchinis
- 2 tbsp. olive oil
- 2tbsp olive oil (too cook zoodles)
- Kosher salt and black pepper (to taste)
- 2 c. Roma tomatoes, seeded and chopped
- 1 c. shredded mozzarella
- 1 tsp. Italian seasoning
- ½ tsp garlic powder
- 2 tbsp. red wine vinegar

Directions

1. Use a spiralizer or a vegetable peel to make noodles out of the zucchini.
2. Heat olive oil in a nonstick skillet (medium heat).

3. Add zoodles, salt, pepper and sauté for 4 minutes.
4. Carefully flip zoodles so that they cook thoroughly.
5. Remove from heat when Zoodles are tender.
6. In a large bowl, combine zoodles, olive oil, seasoning, salt and pepper to taste.Coat zoodles well.
7. Marinate for 10 minutes.
8. Add tomatoes and mozzarella.
9. Sprinkle red wine vinegar over zoodles.
10. Serve immediately.

Nutrition Facts

- Servings: 4
- Amount per serving
- Calories 201
- % Daily Value*
- **Total Fat 13.3g17%**
- Saturated Fat 4.8g 24%
- Cholesterol 19mg6%
- Sodium 235mg10%
- **Total Carbohydrate 10.3g 4%**
- Dietary Fiber 2.9g10%
- Total Sugars 5g
- Protein 12.9g
- Vitamin D 0mcg0%
- Calcium 61mg5%
- Iron 1mg5%
- Potassium 665mg 14%

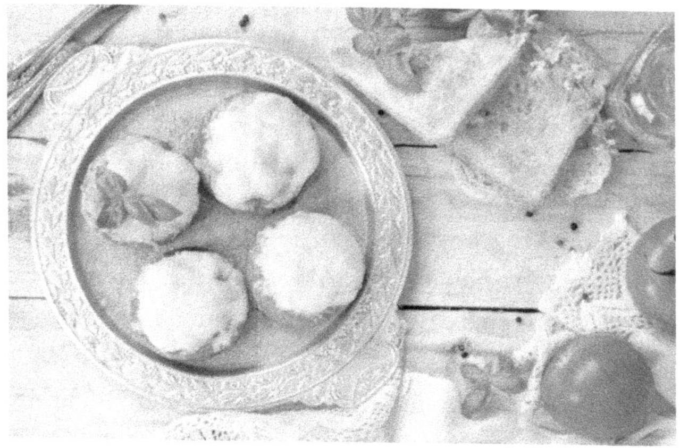

Super Burger Stuffed Tomatoes

- Yields: 4 Servings
- Prep Time: 0 Hours 5 Minutes
- Total Time: 0 Hours 20 Minutes

Ingredients

- 1 tbsp. olive oil
- 1 small red onion, chopped
- 3 cloves garlic, minced
- 1 lb. ground turkey
- 1 tbsp. ketchup
- 1 tbsp. Dijon mustard
- ½ tbsp. mayonnaise
- 4 large tomatoes
- Sea Salt and pepper to taste
- 2/3 c. shredded Colby Jack cheddar
- 1/2 c. shredded iceberg lettuce
- 4 hamburgers sliced pickles

Directions

1. In a skillet over medium heat, cook onion until soft (3 minutes).
2. Add garlic.
3. Add ground turkey and break up into small pieces with a spoon or spatula.
4. Cook ground turkey until there is no pink (5 min)
5. Keep ground turkey on warm heat.
6. Prepare to cut tomatoes by placing them stem down on the cutting board.
7. Without cutting the tomato down to the steam, carefully cut six wedges - stopping before you reach the stem (The tomato needs to stay whole but pliable enough to stuff it).
8. Opening tomato, spoon ground turkey mixture into tomato.
9. Add cheese on top.
10. Add dollops of mustard, ketchup or mayonnaise on top of each tomato (according to your taste favorites).
11. Top with round slices of pickle.

Nutrition Facts

- Servings: 4
- Amount per serving
- Calories 341
- % Daily Value*
- Total Fat 18.5g 24%
- Saturated Fat 3.5g 18%
- Cholesterol 120mg 40%
- Sodium 346mg 15%
- Total Carbohydrate 11.6g 4%
- Dietary Fiber 2.8g 10%
- Total Sugars 6.7g
- Protein 37.8g
- Vitamin D 0mcg 0%
- Calcium 136mg 10%

- Iron 3mg 17%
- Potassium 814mg 17%

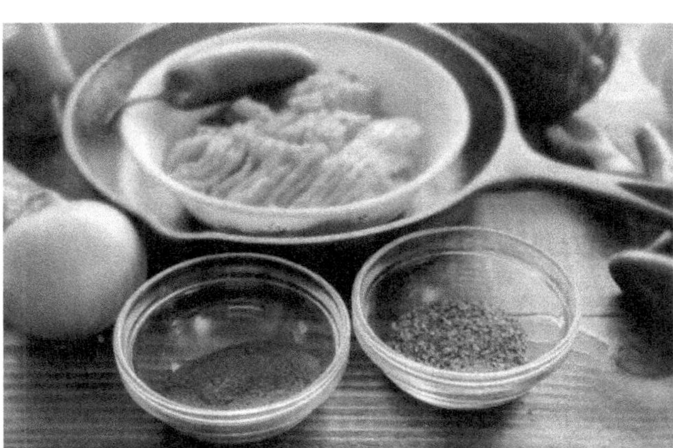

Southwestern Taco Casserole

- Yields: 6 Servings
- Prep Time: 0 Hours 15 Minutes
- Total Time: 1 Hour 0 Minutes

Ingredients

- 1 tbsp. extra-virgin olive oil
- 1/2 white onion, diced
- 2 lb. ground turkey
- 2 tbsp. kosher salt
- Freshly ground black pepper
- 2 tbsp. keto taco seasoning mix (see xyz recipe)
- 2 pickledjalapeño, slices (reserve some slices for garnish)
- 6 large eggs, lightly beaten
- 2 c. shredded cheddar cheese
- 2 tbsp. freshly cilantro leaves

- 1 c. sour cream, for serving (optional)

Directions

1. Preheat Oven to 350°.
2. Brown ground turkey,in large skillet over medium high heat until there is no longer any pink (break up with spoon or spatula as you are browning meat).
3. Add taco seasoning and salt and pepper to taste.
4. Add pickled jalapeños (reserve some for garnish).
5. In a medium bowl, beat eggs.
6. Remove skillet from heat, cool slightly and then add beaten eggs (drain fat is desired and then put back in skillet and add egg mixture).
7. Spread mixture into a 2 quart baking dish.
8. Sprinkle with cheese.
9. Bake for 25 minutes.
10. Sprinkle with cilantro and jalapeños.
11. Top with sour cream.
12. Serve immediately.

Nutrition Facts

- Servings: 6
- Amount per serving
- Calories 624
- % Daily Value
- Total Fat 44.4g 57%
- Saturated Fat 17.6 88%
- Cholesterol 397mg 132%
- Sodium 2812Mg 122%
- Total Carbohydrate 3.4g 1%
- Dietary Fiber 0.2g 1%
- Total Sugars 1g
- Protein 58.4g

- Vitamin D 22mcg 110%
- Calcium 384mg 30%
- Iron 4mg 23%
- Potassium 583mg 12%

~

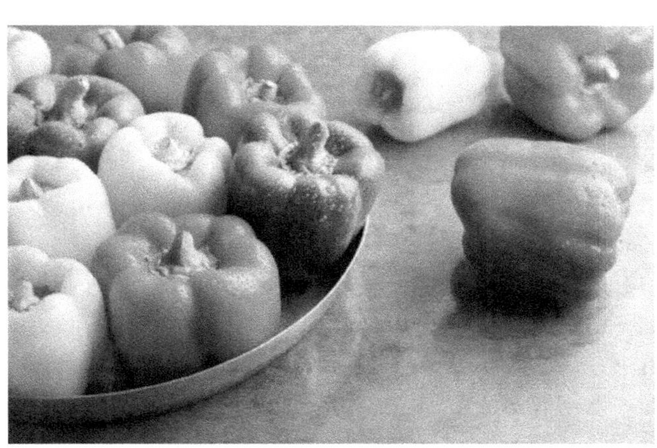

Stuffed Peppers

- Yields: 6 Servings
- Prep Time: 0 Hours 15 Minutes
- Total Time: 0 Hours 35 Minutes

Ingredients

- 1 tbsp extra-virgin olive oil
- 1 c. yellow onion, chopped
- 2 cloves garlic, minced
- 1 lb. ground turkey
- Kosher salt
- Freshly ground black pepper
- 2 tbsp. Chopped cilantro
- 2 tsp. Keto Taco seasoning

- 3 bell peppers, halved (seeds removed)
- ½c. shredded Cheddar
- ½c. Shredded Monterey Jack
- 1 c. Shredded lettuce
- Pico de gallo, for serving*

Directions

1. Preheat oven to 375°.
2. In large nonstick skillet over medium heat, sauté onion until tender.
3. Add ground turkey and breaking up into little pieces, brown until no longer pink.
4. Add Keto taco seasoning, and season with salt and pepper to taste.
5. Turn off heat.
6. Place bell peppers in a 2 quart baking dish, cut side up.
7. Drizzle with olive oil.
8. Season with salt and pepper to taste.
9. Fill each pepper with ground turkey mixture.
10. Add both cheeses to top of bell peppers.
11. Bake for 30 minutes (bell pepper should be tender).
12. Serve immediately.
13. *Pico de gallo -is just chopped tomatoes, onion and cilantro mixed together.

Nutrition Facts

- Servings: 3
- Amount per serving
- Calories 459
- % Daily Value*
- Total Fat 24.3g 31%
- **Saturated Fat 5.1 25%**
- Cholesterol 162mg 54%

- Sodium 449mg 20%
- **Total Carbohydrate 14.6g 5%**
- Dietary Fiber 2.6g 9%
- Total Sugars 8g
- **Protein 52.4g**
- Vitamin D 0mcg 0%
- Calcium 218mg 17%
- Iron 4mg 24%
- Potassium 751mg 16%

~

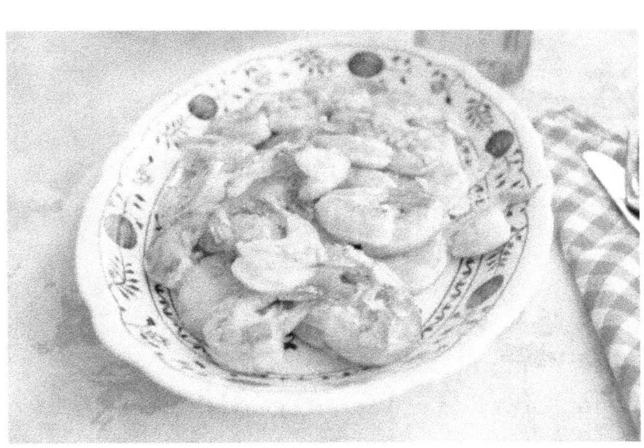

Butter Shrimp

- Yields: 4 Servings
- Prep Time: 0 Hours 5 Minutes
- Total Time: 0 Hours 20 Minutes

Ingredients

- 2 tbsp. extra-virgin olive oil
- 1 lb. shrimp, peeled, deveined, and tails removed
- Sea Salt

- Freshly ground black pepper
- 3 tbsp. butter
- 3 cloves garlic, minced
- 1 1/2 c.tomatoes, chopped
- 3 c. baby spinach
- ½ c. mushrooms, sliced
- 1/2 c. heavy cream
- 1/4 c. freshly grated Romano cheese
- 1/4 c. basil, thinly sliced
- Lemon wedges, for serving (optional)

Directions

1. In cast-iron skillet over medium-high heat, add oil.
2. Add shrimp.
3. Season shrimp with salt and pepper.
4. Cook shrimp for 2 minutes and then flip to the other side for 2 minutes (shrimp should be golden and opaque).
5. Remove shrimp from skillet.
6. Reduce heat and add butter, when melted stir in garlic. Cook for 1 minute.
7. Add tomatoes and cook until heated through.
8. Add mushrooms.
9. Add spinach and cook until it wilts.
10. Stir in heavy cream, Romano cheese and basil.
11. Bring mixture to a simmer and then reduce heat to low.
12. Simmer for 4 minutes.
13. Return shrimp to skillet and combine with mixture.
14. Cook until shrimp is heated.
15. Serve on dish with basil for garnish.
16. Sprinkle with lemon juice if desired.

Nutrition Facts

- Servings: 4

- Amount per serving
- Calories 428
- % Daily Value*
- **Total Fat 29.1g 37%**
- Saturated Fat 14.2g 71%
- Cholesterol 304mg 101%
- Sodium 621mg27%
- **Total Carbohydrate 7.5g 3%**
- Dietary Fiber 1.5g 5%
- Total Sugars 2.2g
- **Protein 34.7g**
- Vitamin D 45mcg 226%
- Calcium 377mg29%
- Iron 2mg 9%
- Potassium 553mg 12%

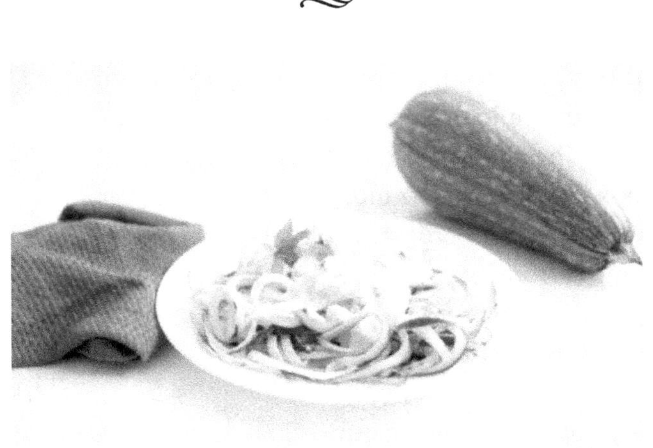

Healthy Alfredo with Bacon

- Yields: 4 Servings
- Prep Time: 0 hours 5 Minutes
- Total Time: 0 hours 20 Minutes

Ingredients

- 1/2 lb. center cut bacon cooked until crispy, chopped
- 2 tbls. Olive oil
- 1 shallot, chopped
- 2 cloves garlic, minced
- ½ cup white grape juice
- 1 1/2 c. heavy cream
- 1/2 c. grated Romano cheese, plus more for garnish
- 1 (16 oz.) container zucchini noodles*
- Sea Salt
- Pepper

Directions

1. Place olive oil in nonstick skillet and heat over medium heat.
2. Add garlic and shallot and cook for 1 minute.
3. Add grape juice and cook until reduced by half.
4. Add cream and bring to a boil.
5. Reduce heat to low and add Romano, stirring.
6. Cook for 2 minutes or more until sauce thickens.
7. Add Zucchini noodles* and combine well .
8. Remove from heat.
9. Sprinkle bacon on top .
10. Serve immediately.

*Make your own following our recipe

Nutrition Facts

- **Servings: 4**
- **Amount per serving**
- **Calories 554**
- **% Daily Value***
- **Total Fat 42.2g 54%**

- Saturated Fat 19.9g **100%**
- **Cholesterol** 137mg **46%**
- **Sodium** 1075mg **47%**
- **Total Carbohydrate** 8.9g **3%**
- Dietary Fiber 1.3g **5%**
- Total Sugars 4.8g
- **Protein** 33.2g
- Vitamin D 23mcg 117%
- Calcium 177mg 14%
- Iron 1mg 3%
- Potassium 387mg 8%

∾

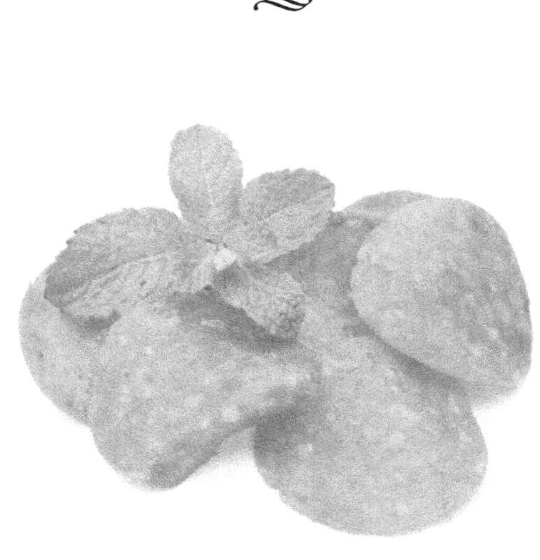

Keto Lunch Box #1

- Yields: 4 Servings
- Prep Time: 0 hours 5 Minutes
- Total Time: 0 hours 10 Minutes

Ingredients

- 3 oz. Pepperoni
- 1 large avocado
- ½ red bell pepper
- 2 oz mozzarella cheese
- ½ cup onion dip

Directions

1. Peel and pit the avocado and then cut into quarters
2. Cut red bell pepper into strips
3. Chop mozzarella into bite-size portions
4. Arrange the vegetables and onion dip into two lunch boxes or a serving platte

*A bento box is perfect for this lunch
Nutrition Facts

- Servings: 2
- Amount per serving
- Calories 745
- % Daily Value*
- **Total Fat 65.9g 84%**
- Saturated Fat 24.7g 123%
- Cholesterol 129mg 43%
- Sodium 1668mg 73%
- **Total Carbohydrate 13.9g 5%**
- Dietary Fiber 7.1g 25%
- Total Sugars 4g
- **Protein 28.3g**
- Vitamin D 6mcg 32%
- Calcium 130mg 10%
- Iron 2mg 11%
- Potassium 741mg 16%

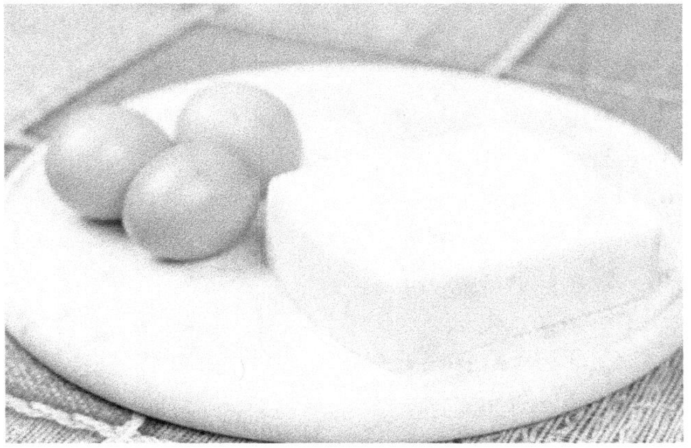

Keto Lunch Box #2

- Yields: 2 Servings
- Prep Time: 0 hours 5 Minutes
- Total Time: 0 hours 10 Minutes

Ingredients

- 3 slices center-cut bacon, cooked until just about crispy
- 2 oz. Mozzarella cheese
- 2 oz Almonds
- 2 hard-boiled eggs

Directions

1. Slice bacon into bite-size pieces
2. cut cheddar cheese into cubes
3. Cut boiled egg into pieces
4. Arrange on a platter or divide into two servings and place in a Bento Box.

Nutrition Facts

- Servings: 2
- Amount per serving
- Calories 462
- % Daily Value*
- **Total Fat 35.4g 45%**
- Saturated Fat 9.5g 47%
- Cholesterol 235mg 78%
- Sodium 905mg 39%
- **Total Carbohydrate 7.6g 3%**
- Dietary Fiber 3.5g 13%
- Total Sugars 2.1g
- **Protein 29.7g**
- Vitamin D 41mcg 205%
- Calcium 329mg 25%
- Iron 2mg 13%
- Potassium 461mg 10%

10
DINNER RECIPES

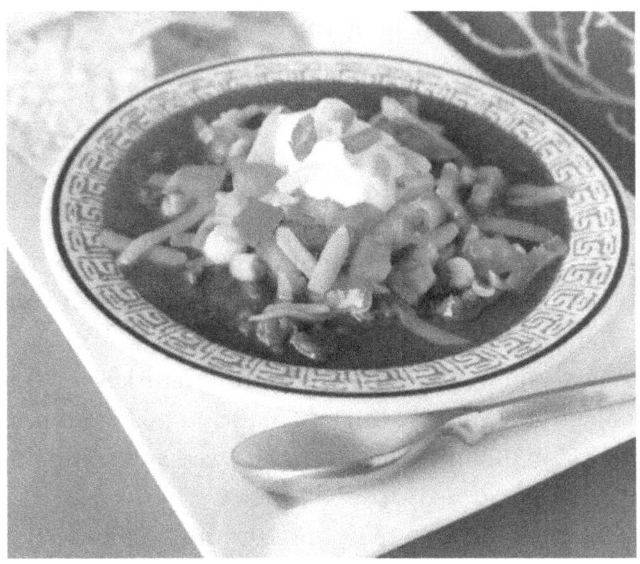

Amazing Chili

- Yields: 8 Servings
- Prep Time: 0 Hours 10 Minutes
- Total Time: 0 Hours 45 Minutes

Ingredients

- 3 slices center cut bacon, cooked
- 1/2 medium white onion, chopped
- 1/2 c. green bell pepper, chopped
- ½ c. orange bell pepper, chopped
- 1/2 c. sliced mushrooms (any variety)
- 2 tbsp. olive oil
- 3 cloves garlic, minced
- 2 lb. ground turkey
- 2 tbsp. homemade taco seasoning*
- Sea salt and pepper to taste
- 2 c. beef broth
- Sour cream, for garnish
- Shredded cheddar, for garnish
- Sliced green onions, for garnish
- Sliced avocado, for garnish
- ½ cup tomatoes, diced, for garnish

Directions

1. In a large Dutch Oven, heat olive oil over medium heat.
2. Add onion, bell pepper and mushrooms and sauté until tender.
3. Remove onion mixture and add ground turkey.
4. Cook ground turkey until browned and no longer pink.
5. Add onion mixture back to Dutch Oven and combine with ground turkey.
6. Add homemade taco seasoning and add salt and pepper to taste combine well.Cook for 3 minutes).
7. Add beef broth to meat mixture and bring to a boil and then turn down the heat and let the chili simmer.
8. Cook for 15 minutes or until the broth is cooked down.
9. Serve in bowls and top with sour cream, bacon crumbles, cheese, green onions and avocado.

Nutrition Facts

- Servings: 4
- Amount per serving
- Calories 745
- % Daily Value*
- **Total Fat 48.1g62%**
- Saturated Fat 10.5g 52%
- Cholesterol 247mg82%
- Sodium 960mg42%
- **Total Carbohydrate 10.7g 4%**
- Dietary Fiber 4.3g15%
- Total Sugars 3.2g
- **Protein 77.2g**
- Vitamin D 63mcg315%
- Calcium 233mg18%
- Iron 6mg33%
- Potassium 1161mg25%

~

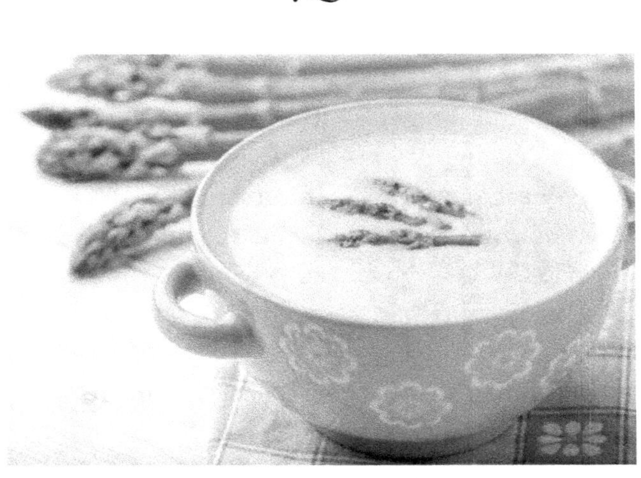

Creamy Asparagus Soup

- Yields: 4 Servings
- Prep Time: 0 Hours 15 Minutes
- Total Time: 0 Hours 40 Minutes

Ingredients

- 2 tbsp olive oil
- 2 cloves garlic, minced
- 2 lb. asparagus, ends trimmed, cut into 1" pieces
- Sea salt and pepper to taste
- 2 c. chicken broth
- 1/2 c. heavy cream, plus more for garnish
- 4 green onions, for garnish

Directions

1. Using a Dutch oven, over medium heat, add olive oil and heat.
2. Add garlic and cook for 1 minute, careful not to let garlic burn.
3. Add asparagus and cook for 5 minutes, season with salt and pepper.
4. Add broth and simmer for 10-12 minutes (don't let asparagus change colors – keep it green but tender).
5. Turn off heat and cool soup for 10 minutes.
6. When cool, pour soup into blender to puree.
7. Return to Dutch Oven and add cream.
8. Let soup warm up – season again with salt and pepper – to your tastes.
9. Garnish with green onions and heavy cream.
10. Serve immediately.

Nutrition Facts

- Servings: 4

- Amount per serving
- Calories 183
- % Daily Value*
- **Total Fat 13.5g17%**
- Saturated Fat 4.7g 24%
- Cholesterol 21mg7%
- Sodium 395mg17%
- **Total Carbohydrate 11.3g 4%**
- Dietary Fiber 5.2g19%
- Total Sugars 5g
- **Protein 8.1g**
- Vitamin D 8mcg39%
- Calcium 83mg6%
- Iron 5mg30%
- Potassium 620mg 13%

~

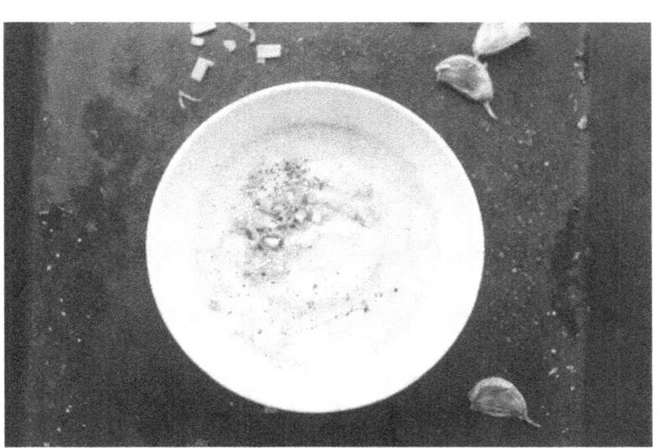

Cheerful Cauliflower Chowder

- Yields: 6-8
- Prep Time: 0 Hours 10 Minutes
- Cook Time: 0 Hours 25 Minutes

- Total Time: 0 Hours 35 Minutes

Ingredients

- 2 tbsp. olive oil
- 1 medium white onion chopped
- 2 carrots, chopped
- 2 stalks of celery, chopped
- Sea salt and pepper to taste
- 3 cloves garlic
- 2 tbsp. Almond flour
- 2 tsp. dried thyme
- 1 head of cauliflower, cut into florets
- 3 cups chicken broth
- 1 c. whole milk
- 2 sprigs of fresh thyme for garnish

Directions

1. In a large saucepan, over medium heat, add olive oil.
2. Add onion, carrots and celery. Cook until onions are translucent and carrots and celery are firm (3 minutes).
3. Add garlic and cook for 1 minute.
4. Stir in almond flour and coat vegetable mix cook for 2 minutes.
5. Add cauliflower and thyme.
6. Add broth and milk slowly stirring.
7. Bring soup to a boil and quickly reduce heat.
8. Simmer until cauliflower is tender (15 minutes).
9. Season with salt and pepper.
10. Ladle soup into bowls.
11. Garnish with fresh thyme sprigs.

Nutrition Facts

- Servings: 4
- Amount per serving
- Calories 127
- % Daily Value*
- **Total Fat 4.1g 5%**
- Saturated Fat 1.5g 8%
- Cholesterol 6mg 2%
- Sodium 684mg30%
- **Total Carbohydrate 15.2g 6%**
- Dietary Fiber 4g14%
- Total Sugars 7.5g
- **Protein 8.1g**
- Vitamin D 24mcg122%
- Calcium 116mg9%
- Iron 1mg8%
- Potassium 537mg 11%

~

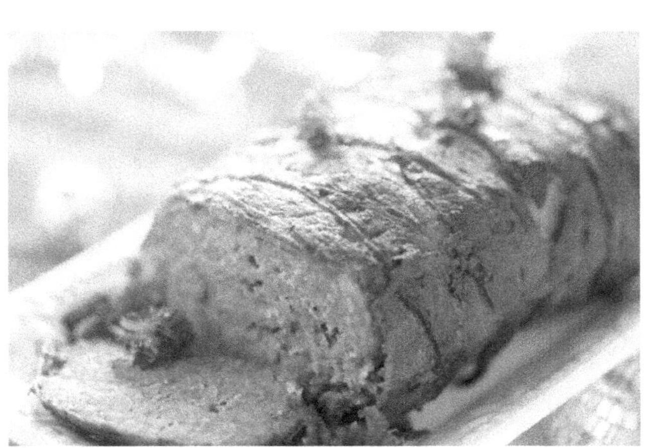

Miracle Meatloaf

- Yields: 6 Servings
- Prep Time: 0 Hours 15 Minutes

- Total Time: 1 Hour 15 Minutes

Ingredients

- Cooking spray
- 1 tbsp.olive oil
- 1 medium white onion, chopped
- 3 cloves garlic, minced
- 2 tbsp. Homemade Taco Seasoning (from earlier part of book)
- 2 lb. ground turkey
- 1 c. shredded pepper jack cheese
- 1/2 c. almond flour
- 1/4 c. grated Parmesan
- 2 eggs
- 1 tbsp. Soy sauce
- Sea salt and pepper to taste
- 6 center cut strips, bacon

Directions

1. Preheat Oven to 400^0.
2. Spray loaf pan with cooking spray.
3. Heat oil in skillet over medium heat.
4. Add onion and cook until translucent (4 minutes).
5. Stir in garlic, taco seasoning, and cook (1 minute).
6. Remove from heat and let cool until you are able to handle it.
7. Use large bowl to combine, ground turkey, onion, cheese almond flour, parmesan, eggs and soy sauce.
8. Shape into loaf and place in loaf plan.
9. Put strips of bacon on top of meat mixture in loaf pan.
10. Cook for 1 hour.
11. Take out at 20 minutes and cover loaf pan with foil so that bacon doesn't get too crisp and burn.

12. Put back into the oven, bake for 30 more minutes (until center is cooked through).
13. Serve immediately.

Nutrition Facts

- Servings: 6
- Amount per serving
- Calories 488
- % Daily Value*
- **Total Fat 32g41%**
- Saturated Fat 6.5g33%
- Cholesterol 170mg 57%
- Sodium 794mg 35%
- **Total Carbohydrate 3.3g1%**
- Dietary Fiber 0.7g 3%
- Total Sugars 1g
- **Protein 38.4g**
- Vitamin D 5mcg 26%
- Calcium 85mg7%
- Iron 3mg14%
- Potassium 356mg 8%

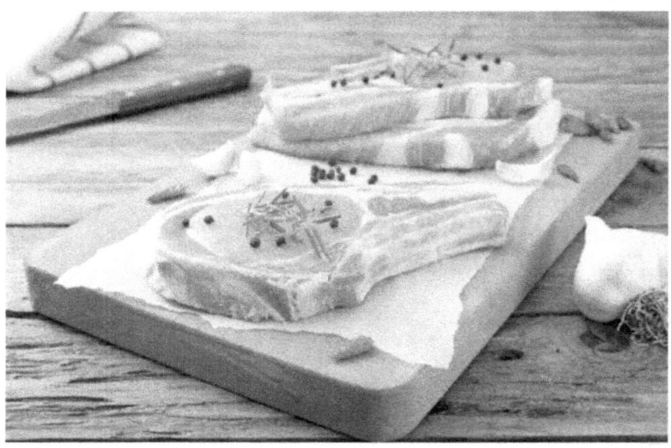

Garlic Pork Chops

- Yields: 4
- Prep Time: 0 Hours 10 Minutes
- Total Time: 0 Hours 30 Minutes

Ingredients

- 4 pork chops
- Salt and pepper to taste
- 2 tbsp. Paprika
- 3 cloves garlic, minced
- 1/2 c. butter, melted
- 1 tbsp. olive oil
- Peppercorns for garnish
- Red peppers for garnish
- Thyme for garnish

Directions

1. Preheat oven to 350⁰.
2. In a small bowl, mix paprika, garlic and butter to make a paste, set aside.

3. Season pork chops with salt and pepper.
4. In an oven-proof skillet, placed over medium-high heat, add olive oil.
5. Add pork chops and cook for 4 minutes on each side.
6. Remove pork chops from heat and add butter paste (leave some butter paste for garnish).
7. Place skillet in the oven and cook for 10-12 minutes until pork chops are done.
8. Take out of oven and lay on serving platter.
9. Brush the rest of the pork with the butter paste.
10. Add peppercorns, thyme and red peppers for garnish.
11. Serve immediately.

Nutrition Facts

- Servings: 4
- Amount per serving
- Calories 493
- % Daily Value*
- **Total Fat 46.4g 60%**
- Saturated Fat 22.5g 113%
- Cholesterol 130mg 43%
- Sodium 220mg 10%
- **Total Carbohydrate 0.8g 0%**
- Dietary Fiber 0.1g 0%
- Total Sugars 0g
- Protein 18.4g
- Vitamin D 16mcg 79%
- Calcium 34mg 3%
- Iron 1mg 4%
- Potassium 291mg 6%

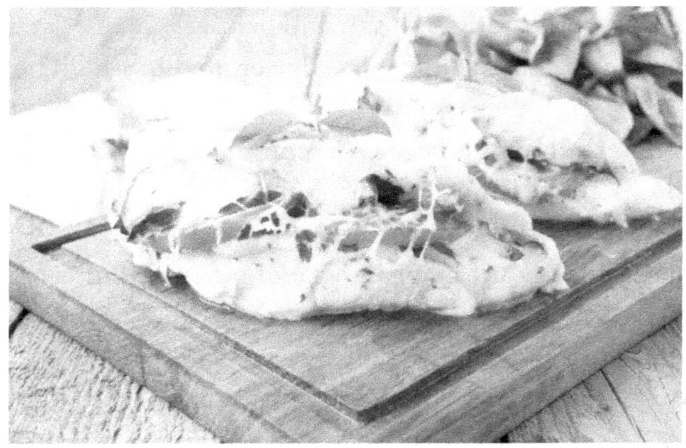

Homestyle Chicken

- Yields: 4 Servings
- Prep Time: 0 Hours 10 Minutes
- Total Time: 0 Hours 35 Minutes

Ingredients

- 2 tbsp. olive oil
- 4 slices center cut bacon, cooked and crumbled
- 4 boneless skinless chicken breasts (about 2 lbs.)
- Sea salt and pepper
- 4 tsp. ranch seasoning
- 1 1/2 c. shredded mozzarella
- Chopped green onions for garnish
- Red pepper for garnish

Directions

1. Season chicken with salt and pepper.
2. Place heavy skillet on medium heat.
3. Add olive oil.
4. Place chicken breasts in skillet and cook for 6 minutes.

5. Turn chicken over and cook for another 6 minutes.
6. Turn down heat to low.
7. Sprinkle ranch dressing seasoning over chicken.
8. Top chicken with mozzarella.
9. Cover skillet and cook for 5 minutes (cheese should melt).
10. Plate chicken on large serving platter.
11. Sprinkle chicken with green onions, red pepper slices and bacon crumbles.
12. Serve immediately.

Nutrition Facts

- Servings: 4
- Amount per serving
- Calories 543
- % Daily Value*
- **Total Fat 23.7g 30%**
- Saturated Fat 6.7g33%
- Cholesterol 201mg 67%
- Sodium 650mg 28%
- **Total Carbohydrate 2.5g1%**
- Dietary Fiber 0.7g 2%
- Total Sugars 0.6g
- **Protein 76.2g**
- Vitamin D 0mcg 0%
- Calcium 57mg4%
- Iron 3mg15%
- Potassium 600mg 13%

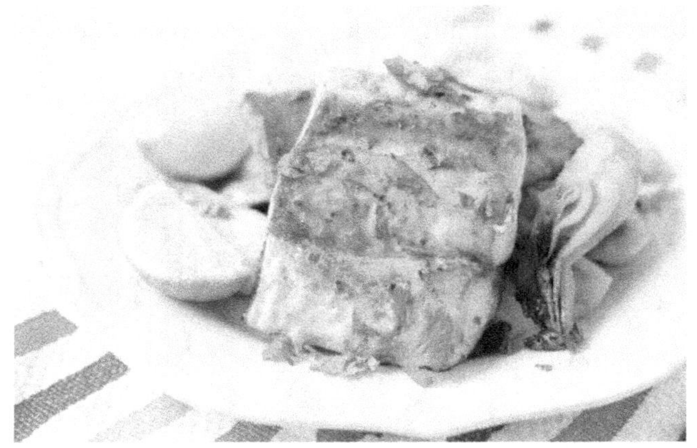

Spicy Mahi Mahi

Ingredients

- 1 tsp. chili powder
- 1/4 tsp garlic powder
- 1/4 tsp. cumin
- 1/8 tsp. onion powder
- 1/8 tsp. cayenne pepper
- tbsp. butter, divided
- 2 tbsp. extra-virgin olive oil, divided
- 4 (4-oz.) mahi-mahi fillets
- Sea salt and ground pepper to taste
- 1 lb. asparagus, cut into bite sized pieces
- 3 cloves garlic, minced
- 1/2 tsp. crushed red pepper flakes (optional)
- 1 lime, sliced
- Zest and juice of 1 lime
- 1 tbsp. freshly chopped cilantro, plus more for garnish

Directions

1. Using 2 tablespoon of butter, mix spices (onion powder,

    cayenne pepper, cumin, chili powder and garlic powder) into a paste (use small bowl to mix).

2. Heat 2 tablespoon of olive oil in large skillet over medium heat.
3. Carefully rub seasoned butter on Mahi Mahi.
4. Place Mahi Mahi into pan and cook 5 minutes on each side.
5. Take out Mahi Mahi and place it on a serving platter.
6. Add 2 tablespoons of butter into skillet.
7. Add asparagus.
8. Add garlic, red pepper flakes and cook for 2 minutes.
9. Stir in lime zest and drizzle lime juice over asparagus.
10. Remove from heat.
11. Place asparagus on plate with Mahi Mahi.
12. Garnish with cilantro.
13. Serve immediately.

Nutrition Facts

- Servings: 4
- Amount per serving
- Calories 386
- % Daily Value*
- **Total Fat 30.2g 39%**
- Saturated Fat 15.6g 78%
- Cholesterol 101mg 34%
- Sodium 262mg 11%
- **Total Carbohydrate 7.5g 3%**
- Dietary Fiber 2.9g 10%
- Total Sugars 2.6g
- Protein 24g
- Vitamin D 16mcg 79%
- Calcium 145mg 11%
- Iron 4mg 20%
- Potassium 270mg 6%

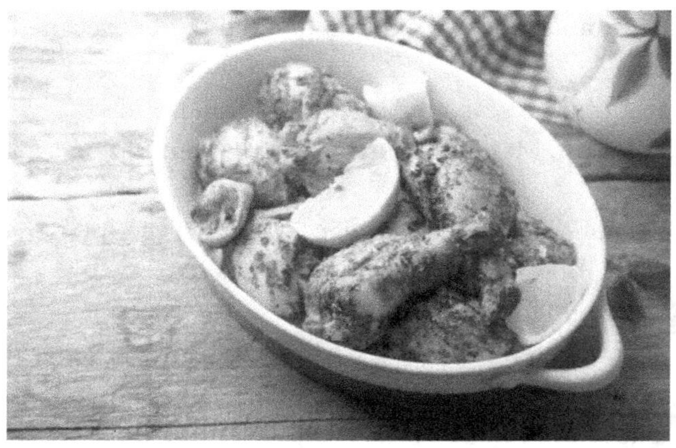

Greek Chicken

- Yields: 4
- Prep Time: 0 Hours 20 Minutes
- Total Time: 0 Hours 50 Minutes

Ingredients

- 2 tbsp. olive oil, divided
- 4 tbsp. lemon juice
- 4 cloves garlic, minced
- 1 tsp. dried oregano
- 1 lb. chicken thighs or drumsticks
- Kosher salt
- Freshly ground black pepper
- ½ cup sliced mushrooms
- 1 zucchini, sliced into half moons
- ½ c. white onions, sliced thin
- ½ cup chicken broth
- 1 lemon, sliced (with peel)

Directions

1. Sprinkle chicken with lemon juice, salt and pepper.
2. Heat large skillet on medium high.
3. Add olive oil and let heat for a few seconds.
4. Place chicken skin side done in skillet.
5. Cook each side of chicken until golden and crispy (10 minutes).
6. Add zucchini, onions and mushrooms.
7. Place lemon slices on top of chicken thighs.
8. Add ¼ cup chicken broth.
9. Cover and let cook until vegetables are tender (15 minutes).
10. Serve immediately.

Nutrition Facts

- Servings: 4
- Amount per serving
- Calories 309
- % Daily Value*
- **Total Fat 15.9g 20%**
- Saturated Fat 3.5g18%
- Cholesterol 101mg 34%
- Sodium 242mg 11%
- **Total Carbohydrate 6.3g2%**
- Dietary Fiber 1.6g 6%
- Total Sugars 2.4g
- **Protein 35g**
- Vitamin D 32mcg158%
- Calcium 45mg3%
- Iron 2mg12%
- Potassium 536mg 11%

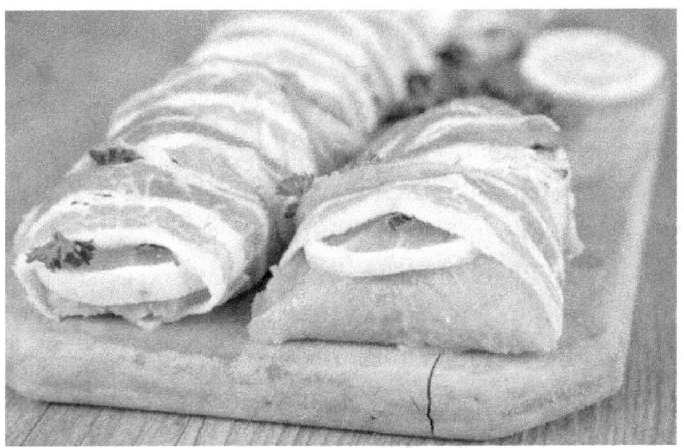

Bacon Wrapped Fish

- Yield: 3
- Prep Time: 0 Hours 5 Minutes
- Total Time: 0 Hours 15 Minutes

Ingredients

- 6 slices center cut bacon
- 3 catfish filets
- Sea salt
- Ground pepper
- 1 tsp. paprika
- Lemon, sliced

Directions

1. Heat oven to 350°.
2. Sprinkle paprika on catfish.
3. Season catfish filet with salt and pepper to taste.
4. Place lemon slices on top of fish.
5. Wrap two slices of bacon around each fish.
6. Bake catfish filet for 20 minutes.

Nutrition Facts

- Servings: 3
- Amount per serving
- Calories 351
- % Daily Value*
- Total Fat 21.2g 27%
- Saturated Fat 6.6g 33%
- Cholesterol 71mg 24%
- Sodium 1124mg49%
- Total Carbohydrate 15.4g 6%
- Dietary Fiber 0.5g 2%
- Total Sugars 0g
- Protein 27.3g
- Vitamin D 0mcg 0%
- Calcium 16mg 1%
- Iron 2mg 11%
- Potassium 291mg 6%

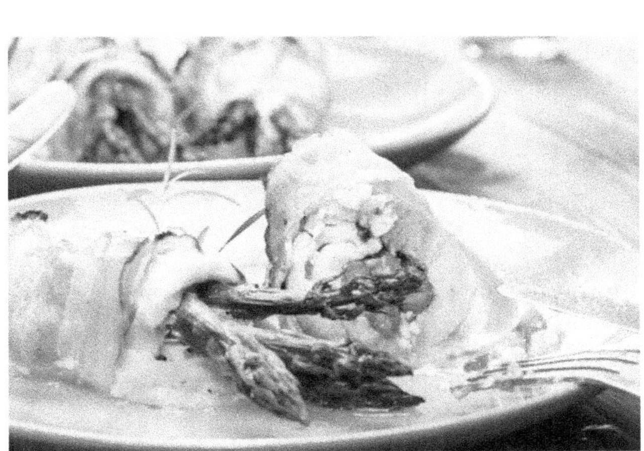

Chicken with Bacon and Asparagus

- Yields: 4
- Prep Time: 0 Hours 5 Minutes
- Total Time: 0 Hours 45 Minutes

Ingredients

- 2 chicken breasts, cut in half
- Sea Salt
- Ground pepper
- 12 asparagus spears
- 8 pieces center cut bacon

Directions

1. Preheat oven to 400°.
2. Place two bacon slices on a jelly roll pan.
3. Lay chicken breast on top of it.
4. Season with salt and pepper to taste.
5. Add asparagus.
6. Finish wrapping bacon around chicken and asparagus (may use toothpicks to secure).
7. Bake for 40 minutes (check chicken for doneness and add 5 minutes if needed).

Nutrition Facts

- **Servings: 4**
- **Amount per serving**
- **Calories 131**
- **% Daily Value***
- **Total Fat 5.7g 7%**
- **Saturated Fat 1.9g 9%**
- **Cholesterol 45mg 15%**
- **Sodium 101mg 4%**
- **Total Carbohydrate 2.8g 1%**

- Dietary Fiber 1.5g 5%
- Total Sugars 1.4g
- **Protein 17.2g**
- Vitamin D 0mcg 0%
- Calcium 24mg 2%
- Iron 2mg 11%
- Potassium 265mg 6%

~

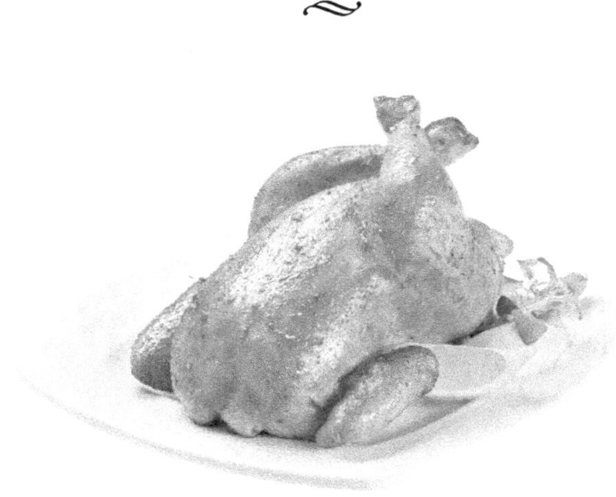

Lemon Roast Chicken

- Yields: 4
- Prep Time: 0 Hours 5 Minutes
- Total Time: 1 Hours 40 Minutes

Ingredients

- 1 roasting chicken
- Sea salt
- Ground pepper
- Paprika
- 1 whole lemon

Directions

1. Preheat oven to 435.
2. Sprinkle salt and pepper over chicken.
3. Empty cavity (if chicken comes with liver etc.).
4. Place chicken in roasting pan.
5. Sprinkle with paprika, salt and pepper.
6. Cut lemon in half.
7. Place lemons in cavity of chicken.
8. Bake for 1 hour or 1/1/2 hr. until juices run clear.

Nutrition Facts

- **Servings:** 6
- Amount per serving
- Calories 178
- % Daily Value*
- **Total Fat** 10.7g
- **14%**
- Saturated Fat 3g 15%
- **Cholesterol 61mg 20%**
- Sodium 58mg 3%
- **Total Carbohydrate 0g 0%**
- Dietary Fiber 0g 0%
- Total Sugars 0g
- **Protein 19.2g**
- Vitamin D 0mcg 0%
- Calcium 10mg 1%
- Iron 1mg 6%
- Potassium 169mg 4%

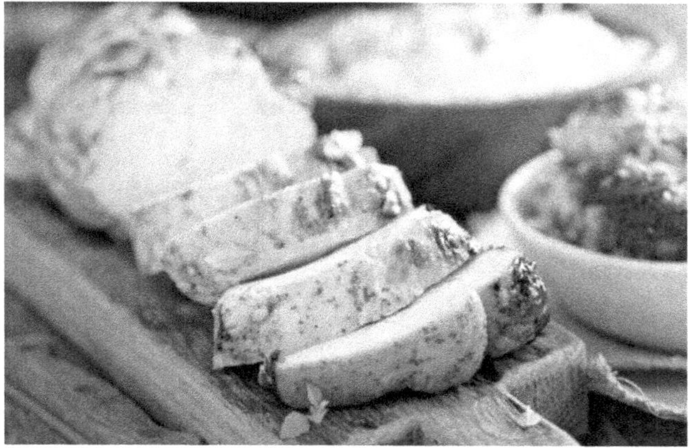

Dinner to Go #1

- Yields: 3 Servings
- Prep Time: 0 Hours 5 Minutes
- Total Time: 0 Hours 10 Minutes

Ingredients

- 6 oz. cooked breast of chicken
- 4 oz. steamed broccoli
- ½ cup cherry tomatoes
- 2 oz. Monterey jack cheese
- 3 oz. ranch dip
- Keto taco spice (in recipe #)
- Salt and pepper to taste.

Directions

1. Season chicken with Keto taco spice to taste.
2. Cut cheese into cubes.
3. Halve cherry tomatoes.
4. Cut broccoli into small bite sized pieces.

5. Arrange everything on a platter or divide into two Bento Boxes.

Nutrition Facts

- Amount per serving
- Calories 419
- % Daily Value*
- Total Fat 18.2g 23%
- Saturated Fat 2.6g 13%
- Cholesterol 156mg 52%
- Sodium 332mg 14%
- Total Carbohydrate 5.6g 2%
- Dietary Fiber 1.3g 5%
- Total Sugars 2.4g
- Protein 57.3g
- Vitamin D 0mcg 0%
- Calcium 64mg 5%
- Iron 2mg 11%
- Potassium 546mg 12%

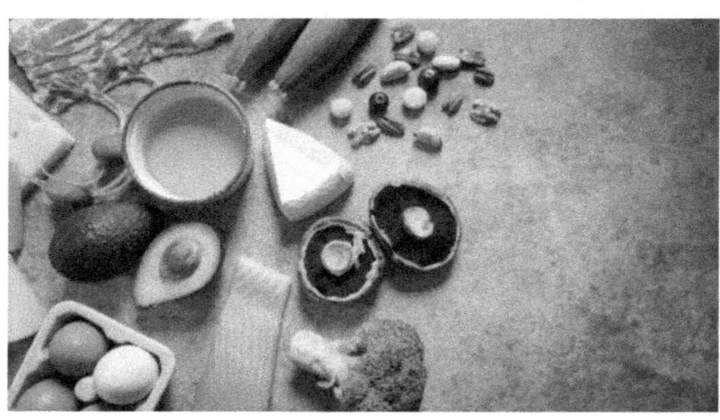

Dinner to go #2

- Yields: 3 Servings
- Prep Time: 0 Hours 5 Minutes
- Total Time: 0 Hours 10 Minutes

Ingredients

- 6 oz, Smoked Salmon
- 4 oz. Mushrooms, sliced
- 1 large avocado
- 4 oz. Steamed broccoli
- 4 oz. blueberries
- 4 oz. almonds

Directions

1. Flake smoked salmon into bite sized pieces.
2. Place guacamole in small bowl.
3. Arrange everything on a platter or divide into two portions and place in Bento box.

~

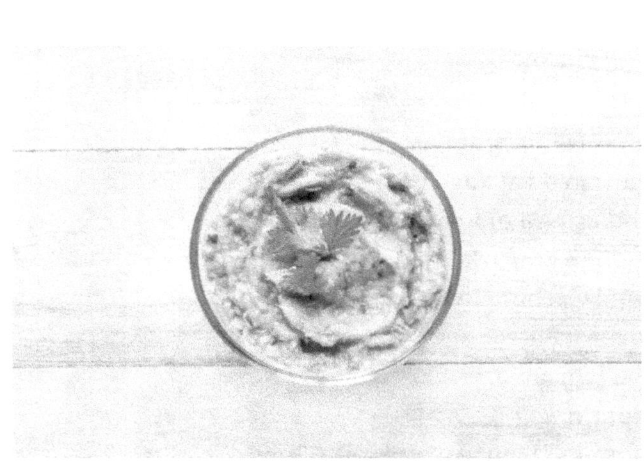

Guacamole Recipe

Ingredients

- 1 large avocado
- ¼ cup tomatoes, diced
- ¼ cup red onion
- 1 small Serrano pepper, seeded and minced*
- 1 half lemon
- Sea salt to taste

Directions

1. Peel and pit avocado.
2. Mash avocado with fork.
3. Mix in tomato and onion.
4. Squeeze juice of lemon.
5. Season with salt.
6. Stir everything together.

Nutrition Facts for Guacamole

- **Servings: 2**
- **Amount per serving**
- Calories 216
- % Daily Value*
- **Total Fat 19.7g 25%**
- Saturated Fat 4.1g 21%
- Cholesterol 0mg 0%
- Sodium 8mg 0%
- **Total Carbohydrate 11.1g 4%**
- Dietary Fiber 7.4g 27%
- Total Sugars 1.8g
- **Protein 2.3g**
- Vitamin D 0mcg 0%
- Calcium 18mg 1%
- Iron 1mg 4%

- Potassium 571mg 12%

Nutrition Facts

- **Servings: 3**
- **Amount per serving**
- **Calories 384**
- **% Daily Value***
- Total Fat 28.1g 36%
- Saturated Fat 2.6g 13%
- Cholesterol 25mg 8%
- **Sodium 154mg 7%**
- **Total Carbohydrate 18.8g 7%**
- Dietary Fiber 8g 28%
- Total Sugars 6.7g
- **Protein 21g**
- Vitamin D 0mcg 0%
- Calcium 140mg 11%
- Iron 3mg 14%
- Potassium 644mg 14%

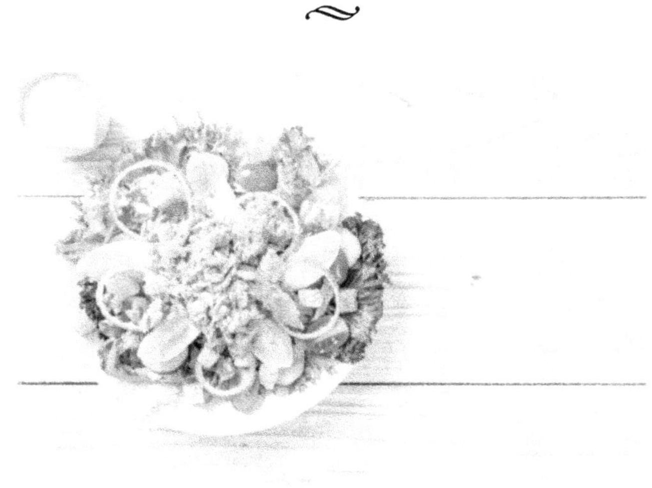

Easy Tuna Fish Delight

- Yields: 2 Servings
- Prep Time: 0 Hours 5 Minutes
- Total Time: 0 Hours 20 Minutes

Ingredients

- 2 3oz packets of tuna
- 1 celery rib, diced
- 3 tbsp. mayonnaise
- ½ c. red onion, chopped
- 1 tbsp. freshly squeezed lemon juice
- 1/4 c. dill relish
- 2 Romaine lettuce leaves
- 3 oz swiss cheese
- 2 pickle spears
- 3 oz. almonds

Directions

1. In a large bowl, place tuna,, celery, onion and dill relish.
2. Add mayonnaise and mix well.
3. Scoop tuna mixture evenly between 2 romaine lettuce leaf.
4. Cube swiss cheese into bite-sized pieces.
5. Arrange everything on a platter or divide into two Bento boxes.

Nutrition Facts

- **Servings: 2**
- **Amount per serving**
- **Calories 618**
- **% Daily Value***
- Total Fat 44.1g 57%

- Saturated Fat 10.8g 54%
- Cholesterol 70mg 23%
- Sodium 1369mg 60%
- **Total Carbohydrate 24.7g 9%**
- Dietary Fiber 8.4g 30%
- Total Sugars 6.3g
- **Protein 35.5g**
- Vitamin D 19mcg 94%
- Calcium 469mg 36%
- Iron 3mg 15%
- Potassium 647mg 14%

11

SNACKS AND SWEETS RECIPES

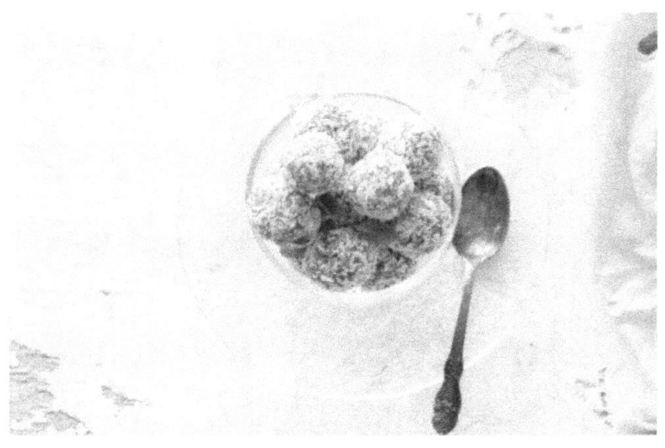

Super Round Carrot Cake

- Yields: 16
- Prep Time: 0 Hours 5 Minutes
- Total Time: 0 Hours 15 Minutes

INGREDIENTS

- 1 (8-oz.) block cream cheese, softened
- 3/4 c. almond flour
- 1 tsp. of any sweetener of your choice (Stevia, Splenda etc.)
- 1 tsp. pure vanilla extract
- 1 tsp. cinnamon
- 1/4 tsp. ground nutmeg
- 1 c. grated carrots
- 1/2 c. Walnuts, chopped
- 1 c. shredded unsweetened coconut

Directions

1. In a mixing bowl, place cream cheese, almond flour, sweetener, cinnamon and nutmeg.
2. Use a hand or stand mixer to mix these ingredients together.
3. Fold in carrots and pecans with wooden spoon.
4. Roll into balls and then cover with shredded coconut.
5. Store in airtight container.

Nutrition Facts

- Servings: 16
- Amount per serving
- Calories 99
- % Daily Value*
- **Total Fat 9.2g 12%**
- Saturated Fat 4.7g24%
- Cholesterol 15mg 5%
- Sodium 54mg 2%
- **Total Carbohydrate 3.3g1%**
- Dietary Fiber 1.1g 4%
- Total Sugars 1.7g
- **Protein 2.5g**
- Vitamin D 0mcg 0%

- Calcium 16mg1%
- Iron 1mg

~

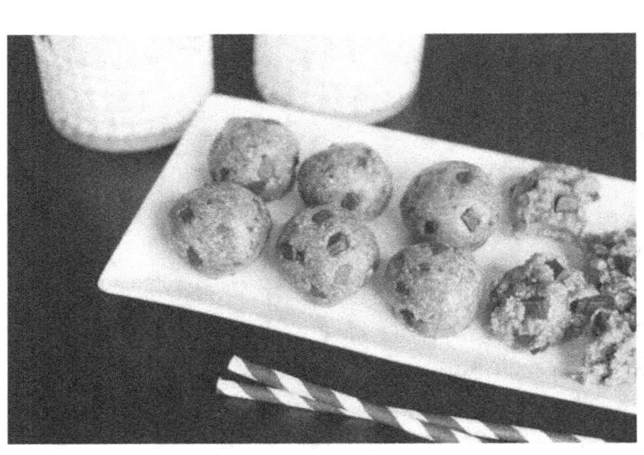

Cookie Dough Balls

- Yields: 30
- Prep Time: 0 Hours 5 Minutes
- Total Time: 1 Hour 5 Minutes

Ingredients

- 1 c. Stevia (or sweetener)
- ½ tsp. vanilla extract
- ½ tsp. sea salt
- 2 c. almond flour
- 2/3 cup dark chocolate chips* (for baking)

Directions

1. In a large bowl, mix butter until fluffy. Use a stand or hand mixer.

2. Add all ingredients EXCEPT for chocolate chips and combine well.
3. While mixer is on, add almond flour slowly until combined.
4. Put mixer aside and fold in chocolate chips.
5. Place bowl in refrigerator for 20 – 25 minutes to chill mixture.
6. Line a cookie sheet with parchment paper.
7. Roll dough into balls and place on parchment paper.
8. Put in freezer for 5 minutes.
9. Take out and enjoy.
10. Put in airtight storage for a week in the refrigerator and one month in the freezer.

***Choose a chocolate chip that contains 70% or more cocoa solids.28 grams of unsweetened chocolate (100%) 3 grams net carbs.**

Nutrition Facts

- Servings: 30
- Amount per serving
- Calories 89
- % Daily Value*
- **Total Fat 4.3g 5%**
- Saturated Fat 0.7g 4%
- Cholesterol 0mg 0%
- Sodium 34mg 1%
- **Total Carbohydrate 9.8g 4%**
- Dietary Fiber 0.8g 3%
- Total Sugars 7.8g
- **Protein 1.8g**
- Vitamin D 0mcg 0%
- Calcium 0mg 0%
- Iron 0mg 0%
- Potassium 0mg 0%

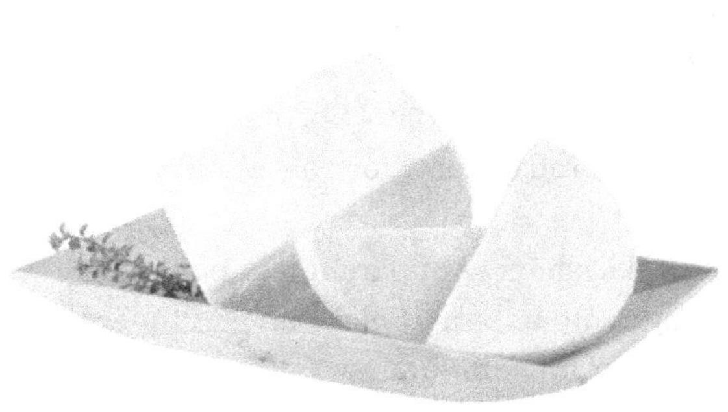

Heavenly Cheese Rolls

- Yields: 4
- Prep Time: 0 Hours 5 Minutes
- Total Time: 1 Hour 5 Minutes

Ingredients

- 8oz. Provolone cheese (or cheese of your choice: edam, cheddar, Swiss, Provolone)
- 2oz. Butter
- ½ pickled jalapeno slices

Directions

1. Place cheese slice on cutting board.
2. Spread butter on cheese slice.
3. Add jalapeño rings at your preference for "heat".
4. Roll cheese up.
5. Enjoy!

Nutrition Facts

- Servings: 4
- Amount per serving
- Calories 301
- % Daily Value*
- **Total Fat 26.6g 34%**
- Saturated Fat 17g 85%
- Cholesterol 70mg 23%
- Sodium 578mg 25%
- **Total Carbohydrate 1.2g 0%**
- Dietary Fiber 0g 0%
- Total Sugars 0.3g
- **Protein 14.6g**
- Vitamin D 8mcg 40%
- Calcium 432mg 33%
- Iron 0mg 2%
- Potassium 82mg 2%

~

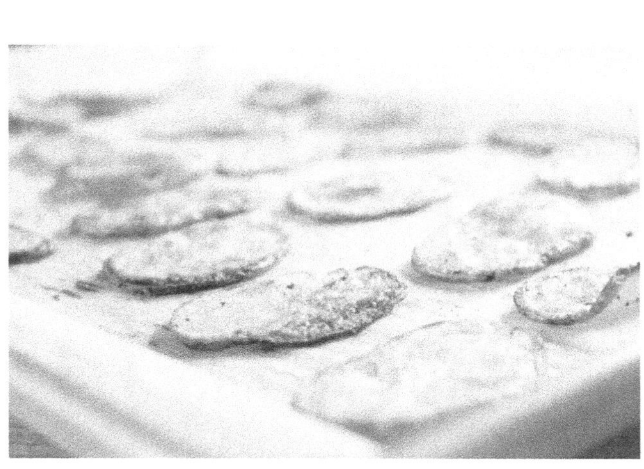

Zesty Avocado Chips

- Yields: 15
- Prep Time: 0 Hours 5 Minutes

- Total Time: 0 Hours 40 Minutes

Ingredients

- 1 large avocado
- 3/4 c. freshly grated Parmesan
- 1 tsp. lemon juice
- 1 tsp. Tabasco
- 1/2 tsp. garlic powder
- Sea salt and pepper to taste

Directions

1. Preheat oven to 325° and line two jelly roll pans with parchment papers.
2. In a large bowl, mash avocado.
3. Stir in Parmesan, lemon juice, garlic powder and Tabasco.
4. Using a teaspoon, scoop out avocado mixture onto baking sheet.
5. Flatten each scoop with back of spatula.
6. Bake until crisp and golden (check every ten minutes 30 minutes total).
7. Cool completely.
8. Serve immediately.

Nutrition Facts

- Servings: 15
- Amount per serving
- Calories 46
- % Daily Value*
- **Total Fat 3.8g 5%**
- Saturated Fat 1.4g7%
- Cholesterol 4mg 1%
- Sodium 55mg 2%

- **Total Carbohydrate 1.4g1%**
- Dietary Fiber 0.9g 3%
- Total Sugars 0.1g
- **Protein 2.1g**
- Vitamin D 0mcg 0%
- Calcium 52mg4%
- Iron 0mg0%
- Potassium 67mg 1%

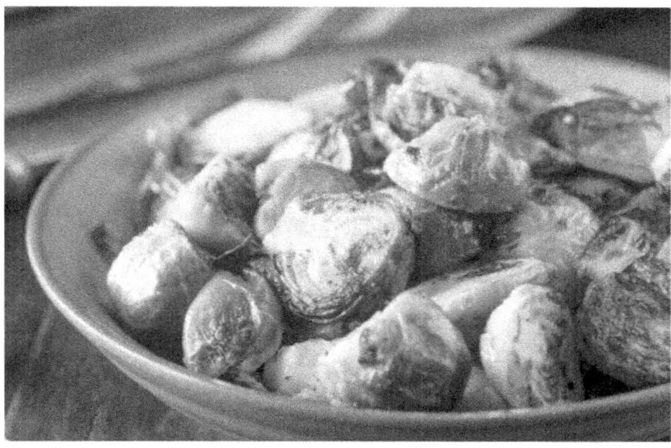

Toasted Brussels Sprouts

- Yields: 2-3 Servings
- Prep Time: 0 Hours 5 Minutes
- Total Time: 0 Hours 25 Minutes

Ingredients

- 1lb. Brussels sprouts, thinly sliced
- 3 tbsp. olive oil
- 4 tbsp. freshly grated Parmesan, plus more for garnish
- 1 tsp. garlic powder

- Sea salt and pepper to taste

Directions

1. Preheat oven to 400⁰.
2. Line jelly roll pan with parchment paper.
3. In a large bowl toss brussels sprouts with olive oil and Parmesan, garlic powder and salt and pepper to taste.
4. Spread carefully on prepared jelly roll pan.
5. Bake 10 minutes and toss.
6. Bake 10 more minutes until crisp and golden.
7. Sprinkle with Parmesan and serve.

Nutrition Facts

- Servings: 6
- Amount per serving
- Calories 108
- % Daily Value*
- **Total Fat 7.9g 10%**
- Saturated Fat 1.8g9%
- Cholesterol 4mg 1%
- Sodium 49mg 2%
- **Total Carbohydrate 7.2g 3%**
- Dietary Fiber 2.9g 10%
- Total Sugars 1.7g
- **Protein 4g**
- Vitamin D 0mcg 0%
- Calcium 66mg5%
- Iron 1mg5%

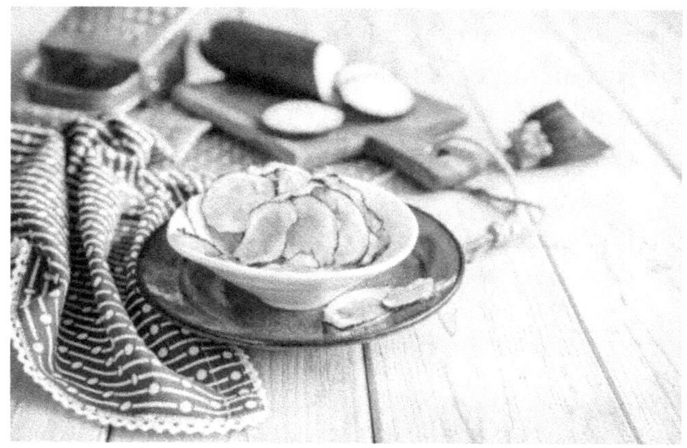

Zucchini Chips

- Yields: 4 Servings
- Prep Time: 0 Hours 10 Minutes
- Total Time: 1 Hour 40 Minutes

Ingredients

1. 2 zucchini, sliced very thinly into coins
2. 1 tbsp. olive oil (for baked version only)
3. 1 tbsp. ranch seasoning
4. 2 tbsp. Parmesan, for garnish
5. Sea salt and pepper to taste

Direction

1. Preheat Oven to 225°Line Jelly Roll pan with parchment paper.
2. Slice zucchini very thing and in rounds (chips).
3. Place on a Jelly Roll pan and use paper towels to get moisture out.
4. Place zucchini and a large bowl and toss with oil, ranch, salt and pepper to taste.

5. Add new parchment paper liner to jelly roll pan.
6. Line zucchini into a single layer on jelly roll pan.
7. Bake until crispy (1hr. 20 min) checking for doneness at ever 20-minute interval.
8. Eat immediately.
9. Store in airtight container.

Nutrition Facts

- Servings: 8
- Amount per serving
- Calories 35
- % Daily Value*
- **Total Fat 2.6g 3%**
- Saturated Fat 0.8g4%
- Cholesterol 3mg 1%
- Sodium 51mg 2%
- **Total Carbohydrate 1.8g1%**
- Dietary Fiber 0.5g 2%
- Total Sugars 0.9g
- **Protein 1.7g**
- Vitamin D 0mcg 0%
- Calcium 39mg3%
- Iron 0mg1%
- Potassium 128mg 3%

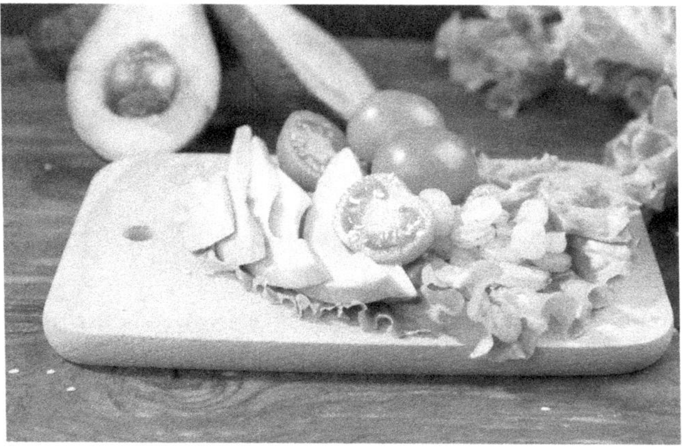

Mexican Shrimp Dip

- Yields: 8 Servings
- Prep Time: 0 Hours 10 Minutes
- Total Time: 0 Hours 25 Minutes

Ingredients

- 1 tbsp. olive oil
- 2 cloves garlic, minced
- 1 tsp. Tabasco
- 1 lb. large shrimp, tails removed
- Sea Salt to taste
- 3 c. tomatoes, seeded and finely diced
- 1/2 c. finely chopped red onion
- 1/2 c. finely chopped cilantro
- 3 Serrano peppers, seeds removed and finely diced (choose to amount according to the heat that you want)
- 1 large avocado, finely diced
- 4 tbsp. fresh lemon juice

Directions

1. In large skillet over medium-high heat, add olive oil and heat.
2. Sprinkle salt and pepper on shrimp.
3. Place shrimp in skillet.
4. Add tabasco sauce.
5. Toss and cook until shrimp is pink and cooked throughout (3 minutes).
6. With a slotted spoon, transfer the shrimp to cutting board.
7. Cool shrimp.
8. Roughly chop the shrimp into bite-sized pieces and place in a large bowl.
9. Add tomatoes, onions, cilantro, Serrano peppers. Lemon juice, and avocado.
10. Season with salt (add more Tabasco if you want more heat).

Nutrition Facts

- Servings: 8
- Amount per serving
- Calories 131
- % Daily Value*
- **Total Fat 6.9g** 9%
- Saturated Fat 1.4g7%
- Cholesterol 81mg 27%
- Sodium 82mg 4%
- **Total Carbohydrate 7.1g3%**
- Dietary Fiber 2.8g 10%
- Total Sugars 2.5g
- **Protein 12g**
- Vitamin D 0mcg 0%
- Calcium 14mg1%
- Iron 0mg2%
- Potassium 318mg 7%

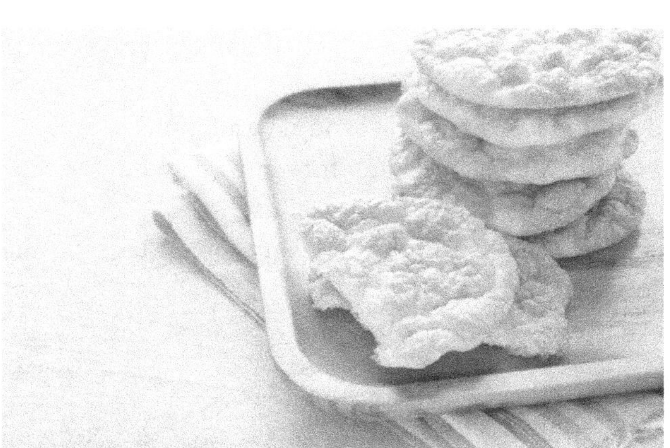

Bagel Cloud Bread

- Yields: 8 Servings
- Prep Time: 0 Hours 10 Minutes
- Total Time: 0 Hours 40 Minutes

Ingredients

- 3 large eggs
- 1/2 tsp. cream of tartar
- 1/8 tsp. sea salt
- 1tsp. minced dried onion
- 1 ½ tsp. ranch seasoning (dry)
- 4 tablespoons cream cheese, softened

Directions

1. Preheat oven to 300°.
2. Line cookie sheet with parchment paper.
3. Separate egg whites from yolks and put them in separate bowls.

4. Add cream of tartar and salt to egg whites and use hand or stand mixer to beat until stiff peaks form (3 minutes).
5. In separate bowl add cream cheese to egg yolks and mix with mixer.
6. Add onions and ranch seasoning and mix.
7. Carefully fold egg yolk mixture into egg whites (keep foamy).
8. Spoon mixture into 8 mounds on prepared cookie sheet and space them 4" apart.
9. Bake until golden 25 to 30 minutes.

Nutrition Facts

- Servings: 8
- Amount per serving
- Calories 46
- % Daily Value*
- **Total Fat 3.6g 5%**
- Saturated Fat 1.7g8%
- Cholesterol 75mg 25%
- Sodium 93mg 4%
- **Total Carbohydrate 0.4g0%**
- Dietary Fiber 0g 0%
- Total Sugars 0.2g
- **Protein 2.7g**
- Vitamin D 7mcg 33%
- Calcium 14mg1%
- Iron 0mg2%
- Potassium 63mg 1%

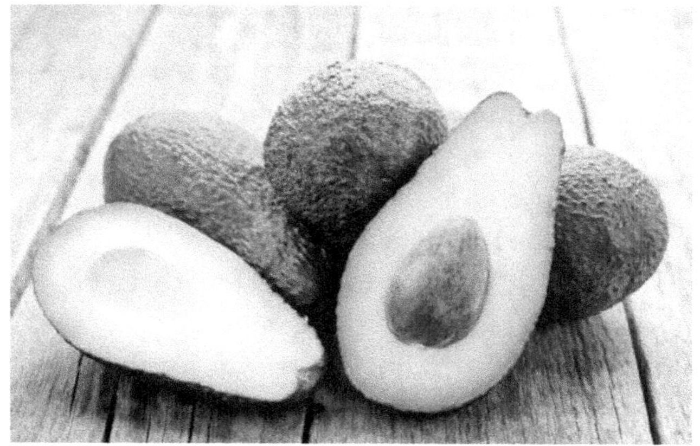

Avocado Bacon Balls

- Yields: 15
- Prep Time: 0 Hours 10 Minutes
- Total Time: 0 Hours 45 Minutes

Ingredients

- 12 slices bacon, cooked
- FOR GUACAMOLE
- 2 large avocados, pitted, peeled, and mashed
- 11 tbsps. cream cheese, softened
- Juice of 1 lemon
- 2 garlic cloves, minced
- 1/4 white onion, minced
- 1 small Serrano pepper (seeded if you prefer less heat), chopped
- 2 tbsp. freshly chopped cilantro
- 1/2 tsp. cumin
- 1/2 tsp. Tabasco (or more to add heat)
- Kosher salt

Directions

1. Line jelly roll pan with parchment paper.
2. Place small skillet over medium heat, sauté onion, Serrano pepper and cumin until onion is translucent and pepper is soft.
3. Remove from heat.
4. In medium bowl mash avocado with fork.
5. Add lemon, salt, onions and pepper and combine.
6. Add cream cheese and combine well.
7. Cover bowl and refrigerate mixture for 30 minutes.
8. Chop bacon and put in shallow dish.
9. With cookie scoop or hands, roll guacamole (avocado) into a ball.
10. Roll ball in bacon.
11. Put on prepared cookie sheet.
12. Eat immediately.

Nutrition Facts

- Servings: 15
- Amount per serving
- Calories 178
- % Daily Value*
- **Total Fat 15.6g 20%**
- Saturated Fat 5.7g28%
- Cholesterol 29mg 10%
- Sodium 399mg 17%
- **Total Carbohydrate 3.2g1%**
- Dietary Fiber 1.9g 7%
- Total Sugars 0.3g
- **Protein 7.1g**
- Vitamin D 0mcg 0%
- Calcium 16mg1%
- Iron 1mg3%
- Potassium 236mg 5%

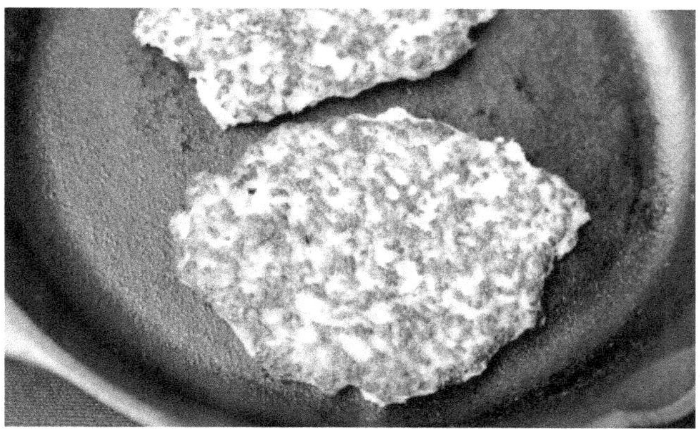

Keto Hash Browns

- Yields: 2 Servings
- Prep Time: 0 Hours 10 Minutes
- Total Time: 0 Hours 25 Minutes

Ingredients

- 2 large eggs
- 1 tsp. garlic powder
- 1/2 tsp. kosher salt
- 1/8 tsp. ground black pepper
- 2 c. shredded cabbage
- 1/4 small white onion, thinly sliced
- 1 tbsp. olive oil

Directions

1. In a large bowl, beat eggs.
2. Add garlic powder, salt and pepper.
3. Add cabbage.
4. Toss together well.

5. Heat the oil in a large skillet (medium high heat).
6. With a hand make a patty (divide mixture into 4).
7. Place patties in skillet.
8. Flatten with back of spatula.
9. Cook patties until they are golden on each side (3 minutes per side).
10. Serve immediately.

Nutrition Facts

- Servings: 4
- Amount per serving
- Calories 79
- % Daily Value*
- **Total Fat 6g 8%**
- Saturated Fat 1.3g6%
- Cholesterol 93mg 31%
- Sodium 332mg 14%
- **Total Carbohydrate 3.2g1%**
- Dietary Fiber 1.1g 4%
- Total Sugars 1.7g
- **Protein 3.8g**
- Vitamin D 9mcg 44%
- Calcium 29mg2%
- Iron 1mg4%
- Potassium 108mg 2%

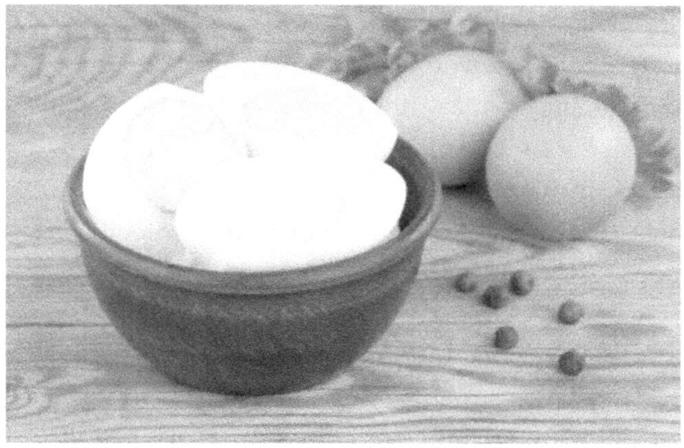

Hard-Boiled Eggs

- Yields: 12
- Prep Time: 0 Hours 5 Minutes
- Total Time: 0 Hours 20 Minutes

Ingredients

- 12 large eggs
- Water

Directions

1. Place eggs in a large saucepan and cover with an inch of water, over medium heat.
2. Bring water to a boil.
3. Remove saucepan from heat.
4. Cover pot and wait (11 minutes).
5. Drain water.
6. Add eggs to ice water for 2 minutes so that .they are easier to peel.

Tips

- Older eggs peel more easily
- Remember to set your timer
- Transfer eggs to ice water right away

Chapter Summary

The best thing you can do for yourself is to cook delicious and healthy food.

- Eggs are very good for you again
- Avocados are a super food
- Don't be afraid to add and change to your meal plan with these recipes

In the next chapter you will learn how to record your progress on simple worksheets.

PART III

TRACKING PROGRESS AND FAQS

12

RECORDING YOUR PROGRESS

The Keto Journal

If buying meters and strips does not appeal to you, there is another choice: the keto journal. A good indicator of how the Keto diet is working for you. These are the types of crucial details, that can show your Keto diet progress.

Paying special attention to the amount of fat, protein and carbs that you are eating can take your diet to a winning level. Further, if you record your energy level daily, you will be able to determine if you need to change your meal or exercise plan. Tracking your energy level and well-being can help you to know if you have reached a state of ketosis. Recording what you eat daily can become a routine that is quick and painless.

The worksheets

Keto Diet Plan	
Date started:	Date:
Present Weight:	Loss/Gain:
Target Weight:	Monthly Progress:
BMI:	

Reason(s) for Starting the Keto diet:
Target Macronutrients: (grams)
Fat:
Carb:
Protein:

Goals:	Action Plans:
1.	
2.	
3.	
4.	
5.	

Keto diet Accomplishments

Before Picture	After Picture

13

FAQS AND CHEAT SHEET

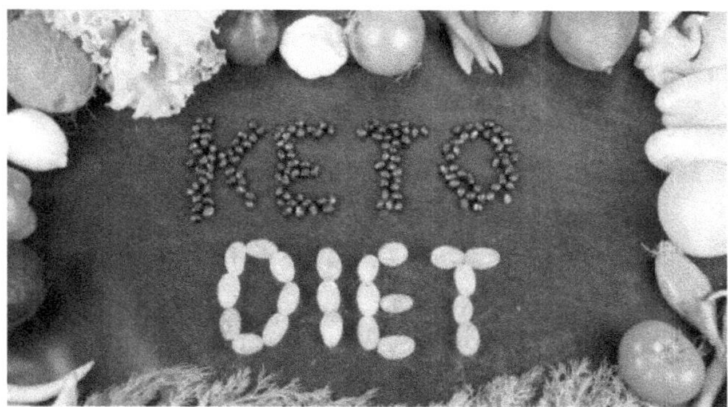

FREQUENTLY ASKED QUESTIONS

By the time you finish reading this book, you will have a clear vision of the Keto diet.What's more, you will have a meal plan, recipes and shopping lists to use on your Keto journey.

However, there are questions that can stump a person at the beginning of a journey.Sometimes the beginning of a journey can feel like it is totally uphill. Here are some frequently asked questions and answers that will help level your path.

. . .

Is The Keto Diet safe?

Developed and tweaked by doctors over the course of almost 100 years, the Keto diet is pretty safe. However, here are some circumstances that need additional planning and/or adjustments

Are you diabetic and on insulin? If you are, it is important that in the beginning, you are very aware of the changes that will be occurring when you consume foods that help you to decrease your blood sugar level. If you do not adjust your medications such as insulin, you might develop a dangerously low blood sugar. Test your blood sugar frequently and share your results with a physician or health professional who is an expert in diabetes and low-carb diets.

Eating foods that will lower your blood pressure is a good thing but not monitoring your dose of high blood pressure medication can lead to feeling weak, tired or dizzy. If your blood pressure goes below 120/80, consult your physician about adjusting the dose of your medication.Again, you might need to find a health professional that is familiar with low-carb diets.

If you are breastfeeding, consult a lactation consultant or health care professional who is familiar with low-carb diets. You are in charge of your baby's nourishment so it is very important that you pay attention to yours. Increasing your carb intake to 50g instead of the standard 25g is usually what is recommended. This doesn't mean you can have fries and a shake. Instead, choose something healthy and on your Keto diet like adding three large fruits per day.

Is It Hard to Know When You've Reached The State of Ketosis?

There are three signs that can be a signpost that you have reached the state of ketosis:

1. Diminished appetite and improved energy levels
2. Increased urination and thirst
3. The appearance of fruity-smelling breath (keto breath)

Remember, if you don't want to depend on signposts, you can use blood meters, breath analyzers and urine strips to determine whether you've reached a state of ketosis.

What Foods Are Best to Avoid When You Are on The Keto Diet?

- Potatoes
- Fruits that are high in sugar like bananas
- Pasta
- White rice
- Beer
- Bread made with white flour or other refined flours
- Soda
- Chocolate bars
- Donuts
- Candy

What Can You Drink on The Keto Diet?

- Water
- Coffee
- Tea
- Red Wine
- Coconut Water
- Vegetable juice

Can You Use Artificial Sweeteners on The Keto Diet?

Drinking a beverage with artificial sweeteners is a lot better than drinking one high in sugar.However, you've got to keep in mind that most studies on the safety of artificial sugar and its impact on our bodies is done by the beverage companies. Not all but a significant number of them. The long-term impact of artificial sweeteners has not been established.

Reasons to avoid artificial sweeteners:

1. They diminish your ability to taste the natural sweetness and flavors of your food and drinks
2. Sweeteners such as Sucralose do affect your blood glucose and insulin response and can add(impact)(effect) to fat storage.

Chapter Summary

- The most important key to success is to track your daily progress
- It is important to adjust your medications with the help of a medical professional, while you are on the Keto diet.
- It's good to add healthy food to your diet versus food not on the Keto diet.
- Be wary of artificial sweeteners

In the next chapter I will share with you some final thoughts.

14

FINAL WORDS

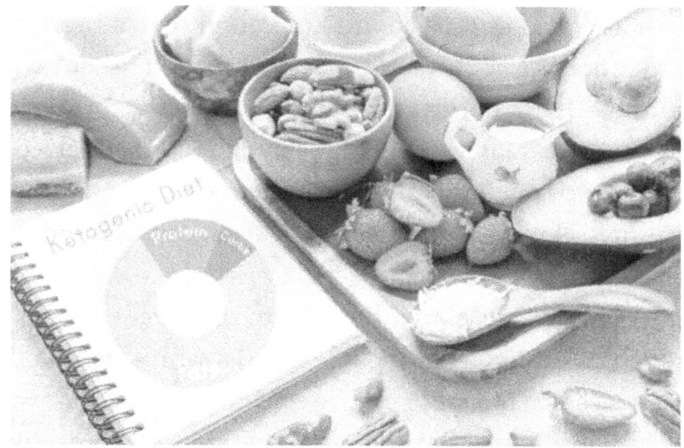

THE KETO DIET IS THE BEST DIET IN THE WORLD. YOU GET TO ADJUST IT and tailor the diet to fit your needs. You get to eat instead of starving yourself. Plus, it has been around for almost a hundred years. What's not to like about the Keto diet?

I would like to leave you with some tips that made my Keto Journey a little bit easier.

. . .

Keto Diet Apps and Websites

The internet has so much information, that it would be a great loss not to further your knowledge about this wonderful diet. There are apps that offer recipes, food gram amounts and Keto Calculators that can really help you to learn more about macronutrients.

It really helps not only to know how many grams of fat, carbs and protein you personally need, but also to learn the gram content of the food you are going to eat. The more you learn about the Keto diet, the more successful you will be. That has been the driving motivation for the creation of this book.

Rehab Your Kitchen and Spend More Time There

Now is the time to spend more time in your kitchen. Reorganize and get rid of all the foods that are harmful to your health. Pantry staples such as bread and pasta are not going to be a big part of your lifestyle anymore. Restock your pantry with foods that are going to add to your health not detract from it.

I started not to fear my kitchen anymore as the place where I committed most of my food "sins". The Keto diet gave me a chance to re-acquaint myself with foods that I had been out of touch with for a long time.

A big part of my success with the Keto diet was wanting to spend more time in my kitchen cooking. I learned a whole new way of cooking. I started to shop for foods that were not processed or made with chemicals and additives that had the potential of being harmful to my health. Since I was spending more time in my kitchen, I spent less time in drive-thru lines and pizza parlors.

Learn to Love Water

When you are burning fat for energy, your need for water increases. I was a big fan of diet soda. I started and ended my day with a big glass filled with the bubbly stuff. Then one day, I didn't feel so good and the only thing that made me feel better was drinking more water. I began to reach for water instead of soda. I bought pitchers that had a special compartment to infuse water. My body thanked me and I had a better feeling about my health and well-being.

No Longer Focused on Weight

There were days when I found it really hard to plan my meals and get enough macronutrients in the right proportions. Yet every time I focused on keeping my carb intake lower, my Keto diet choices just fell into place. The Keto diet is more than a low-carb diet and the more I began to understand that, the better I felt. I changed from focusing on my weight and how many calories I had to omit from my diet; and instead, I learned to focus on getting the right amount of macronutrients in my meal plan.

Reach Out for Support

When I realized that I was not the only one on the Keto diet, I found more motivation to follow my meal plan. There are groups on the internet and in real life that meet to talk about the Keto diet. So many people have had success with this. And sharing their success with you makes the whole journey so much more satisfying. As you progress, you will also enjoy sharing your successes with others. So find a group or a forum where you can learn and share.

Tracking Your Progress

The best thing I ever did for myself was track my progress on the Keto diet. It is good to utilize the different tests that can tell you when you have reached a state of ketosis. However, at some point in your progress, the tests, for various reasons, are not going to be as accurate as they were before. That's where your Keto Journal becomes so important. Writing down and capturing little snapshots of the way you feel during and after your meals is so important. You will begin to see patterns and signs that will become sign posts of your progress and success

Becoming a Planner

It's not just your meals that need to be planned but also your future lifestyle. I used to focus all my celebrations and milestones around eating. If something great happened to me, I would celebrate it with food. When I was well into my Keto diet and felt satisfied with what the Keto lifestyle had to offer, I began to see that there is a whole different world out there. My celebrations stopped being centered around food.

I planned to succeed instead of planning to fail.I stayed away from restaurants that didn't have healthy choices. I invited friends to a fun afternoon at my local park to share and celebrate the milestones in my life. Planning not only your meals but your activities is a sure way to be a winner on the Keto diet.

The Best is Yet to Come

Making the decision to follow the Keto diet is a big deal. You are changing the way your body functions. Yes, there are going to be days when the changes that are happening in your body make you uncomfortable. Yet I am confident that you will experience the health and well being that I found on my Keto Journey.

The fact that you have made the choice to do something about your health is a major conduit for experiencing the best that your body has to offer. Sometimes it takes drastic change to get you to the places you were meant to go. Remember, as you start on your Keto Journey that the best is yet to come.

Final Tips

Always keep in mind the Keto diet food Pyramid and make your food choices accordingly. A suggestion for gram count in the Keto diet is the following:

- Fat 163 grams
- Protein 95 grams
- Carbs 25 grams

(Based on a 2000 calorie a day diet)

You need at least a 20% deficit of calories to lose weight. Remember to always drink your water!

Thank you very much for choosing this book. I wish you all the best!

Image Credit: Shutterstock.com

9 781692 982812